# 375 ESSENTIAL OILS AND HYDROSOLS

JEANNE ROSE

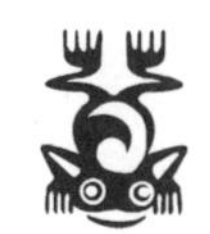

Frog, Ltd.
Berkeley, California

*375 Essential Oils and Hydrosols*


Published by Frog, Ltd.

Frog, Ltd. books are distributed by
North Atlantic Books
P.O. Box 12327
Berkeley, California 94712

Cover and book design by Andrea DuFlon
Printed in the United States of America

Distributed to the book trade by Publishers Group West

**Library of Congress Cataloging-in-Publication Data**

Rose, Jeanne, 1937-
375 essential oils and Hydrosols / by Jeanne Rose.
p. cm.
ISBN 1-883319-89-7 (alk. paper)
1. Essences and essential oils. I. Title. II. Title: Guide to three hundred seventy-five essential oils and hydrosols.
TP958 .R77 1999
661'.806--dc21 98-48682
CIP

3 4 5 6 7 8 9 / 03

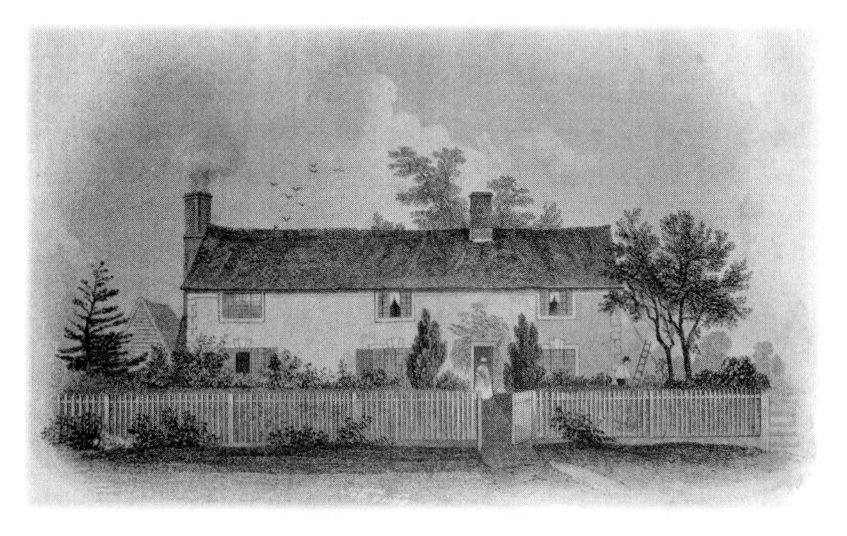

*To all the readers everywhere*
*who by reading my books*
*have supported and*
*nourished my endeavors.*

## Cautions

1. Keep essential oils out of your eyes.
2. Dilute essential oils before use.
3. Identify essential oils by their Latin binomial, part of plant used, variety, and chemical type.
4. Always check your essential oils for color, scent, viscosity, and (sometimes) taste.

Essential oils are volatile and highly concentrated. Do not use essential oils on candles or light bulbs.

## Editor's Note

All plants and essential oils, like all medicine, may be harmful and dangerous if used improperly: if they are taken internally when prescribed for external use, if they are taken in excess, or if they are taken for an undue amount of time, allergic reactions and unpredictable sensitivities or illnesses may develop. It is also important to take into consideration that the strength of wild herbs and various essential oils varies depending on terroir; therefore, knowledge of their growing conditions and distillation methods is helpful. Be sure your herbs are fresh and whole and your essential oils are properly stored. Do not contaminate essential oils with foreign objects like rubber droppers, as they will dissolve in and destroy the essential oil. Keep conditions of use as sterile as possible.

We do not advocate, endorse, or guarantee the curative effects of any of the substances in this book. We have made every effort to ensure that any botanical presented in this book that is dangerous or even potentially dangerous has been identified as such. When you use the plants and their essential oils, recognize their potency and use them with care. Medical or Holistic consultation with a Certified Aromatherapist is recommended.

The botanical names listed under each plant does not always refer to one species only but may refer to others which have been recognized as substitutes in herbal and aromatic medicine.

Please note that in this book the names of plants and their essential oils used therapeutically in herbal or aromatic therapy are capitalized, following ancient tradition.

# Acknowledgements

I wish to acknowledge what I believe to be the three most important books on essential oils. These books helped me tremendously in the creation of *375 Essential Oils and Hydrosols.*

*Perfume and Flavor Materials of Natural Origin*
by Steffen Arctander

*L'aromatherapie exactement*
by P. Franchomme and Dr. Daniel Pénoël

The six volume set of *The Essential Oils*
by Ernest Guenther, Ph.D.

# Contents

*List of Tables*

# Foreword

Ah, 1998! When one procreational/recreational drug, Viagra, reportedly killed 150 Americans (130 reported by CNN on November 25, 1998)! When *Time* magazine features alternative medicine on the cover! When the *Journal of the American Medical Association* (*JAMA*) devoted a whole issue to alternative Medicine! When the *New England Journal of Medicine* criticized Saw Palmetto for working and *JAMA* criticizes garlic for not working. In 1997, they lambasted the "dangers" of herbal medicine while forgetting about the numbers in their own pages; "140,000 Americans Killed by FDA-Approved Drugs in the US." (*JAMA,* 1998). In one recent decade, more than half the new FDA approved drugs had to be recalled permanently (or recalled and re-labeled) because of side effects not anticipated by the $500-million study it now takes to prove a new synthetic drug "safe" and efficacious. In spite of this, physicians, who average less than ten minutes with each of their patients, wonder why more Americans are turning to gentler herbal medicines. Drugs are killing thousands of us. Herbs are helping thousands of us.

Yes. The Herbal Revolution was launched back in Santa Cruz in the early 1970's, where I first met Jeanne Rose. It has marched relentlessly on, leading us into the new millennium. New Age herbs—cheaper, safer, and gentler—have slipped into the pharmacies and HMOs, side by side with synthetic pharmaceuticals. It is a consumer driven revolution, this Herbal Revolution. Yes, Jeanne and I enjoyed sunny Santa Cruz in this formative period of the Herbal Revolution. *La 'Grande Dame'*,* Jeanne Rose and the *herbalbum*, Jim Duke, were among many luminaries there launching the momen-

*Editor's note: Jeanne Rose was known for the publication of the first herbal book, *Herbs & Things,* the first and very popular herbal of the New Age in 1972.

tous revolution. It was my herbal coming out, a closeted herbalist, working with the Medicinal Plant Laboratory of the very conservative USDA. I recall Jeanne's passionate talk, delivered to an outdoor audience. She was herbally active for both positive and negative reasons: negative because chemicals had nearly disabled her lungs, and positive because she had seen the light of the gentler alternative medicines.

Given the choice between an herbal and a pharmaceutical alternative, I'll take the green. In my 69th year, 1998, I've taken a total of seven Advil© tablets, my cumulative synthetic drug consumption for the year. Granted, I've taken several herbs, though only one religiously—celery seed, an herbal alternative to allopurinol. I have been more depressed by the disheartening mortalities in the miniprint on the flip side of the pharmaceutical drug industry than impressed by the quality of the sponsored science in their megaprint. I can name several pairs (herbal alternative/competing pharmaceutical) where the pharmaceutical has killed and the herb has not. Not only am I enjoying good health with my herbal preventative and curative medicines; I am growing them, harvesting them in fields and forests, and spending more than the HMO standard 6 minutes with my green physician, my temple, the forests, with all its green spirits.

Like Jeanne, I have developed a growing respect for Traditional Chinese herbal medicine, Ayurvedic herbs, Native American herbs (North, Central and South American), and am particularly impressed with the power of the aromatic plants and their essential oils. Essence, of course means spirit, and the spirits of the plants are, literally and figuratively, the volatile molecules by which we unconsciously identify many plants. Our genes already know the friendly aromatic plants, if our parents, grandparents, or ancestors sniffed or ingested them.

As we languished on the sunny slopes of Santa Cruz, who could have anticipated that one of the aromatic compounds our ancestors had known, methyl salicylate, was used by the plants to communicate with one another. When one plant is attacked by an herbivore, it converts some of its relatively non-volatile salicylates to volatile methyl salicylate, a Paul Revere molecule which wafts off to the next individual plant to alert it that the herbivores are coming. On every continent humans have learned independently the medicinal attributes of this messenger molecule. It is part of the essence of many plants, though often below the threshold at which our noses can detect the salutary spirit. This morning, my knee has the characteristic wintergreen aroma, alleviating the pain of an arthritic ex-jogger's knee which pushed the lawnmower too hard yesterday.

I feel sorry for those anosmic people I know, unable to detect the molecular messages of the fragrant flowers and herbs. But, whether I am traveling with Shuar Shamans, Sinese Scientists, Seminole Swamp-runners, or Sinai Specialists, I note that all inquiring minds, when asked about the identity of an herb, first look for the morphology, the overall appearance; then smell, for the volatile biochemistry, and sometimes even taste, for the less volatile molecules, gathering the various clues that enable us all to identify plants. Some seem even to have a sixth sense to understand the innate healing ability of the herb with no prior experience of the herb. Such is the case of my shamanistic healer, my Cocama Indian friend in Peru, Antonio Montero Pisco. He describes humanoid essences in the plants, with a characteristic suite of spirits for each species of plant. Big spirits, little spirits, good and evil, tall and short, thin and fat, male and female, hot and cold, black and white, yin and yang, etc, etc... Is he seeing the thousands of homeostatic equilibrating chemical reactions constantly taking place in living plants and animal? Homeostatic equations keep us in balance, within reason! Taking a balanced (read checks and balances, antagonisms and synergistic mixes of thousands of chemicals) herbal medicine is less likely to upset the balance of the homeostatic patient, with his or her thousands of simultaneous homeostatic equilibrating chemical reactions constantly in play. Less likely to upset than the solitary synthetic silver bullet, which may indeed act faster and stronger, both on and off target, hence accompanied by faster, more frequent and more frightening side effects.

I don't see the spirits that Antonio sees. But then again, he is often aided by molecular messengers. Atropine, n,n-dimethyltryptamine, harmine-oxide, harmine, harmaline, myristicin, nicotine, scopoletin, and scopolamine, e.g., molecules that open the mind, albeit dangerously, to see his spirit world. He sees human spirits. I, poor chemist that I am, have visions of molecular models appearing as an orgy of black, white, red and green pool balls getting it on. I know my point of view is not real. I don't know about his. Perhaps when I peek into the soul of the ceiba tree with the sustenance of the soul vine (essence again), I'll see that the Shaman and I are seeing the same thing, from different paradigms. My energized poolballs and his humanoid spirits are the same, the reason we hold up a plant and sniff, the essence of the plant.

Who among us would have guessed in Santa Cruz that the metabolites of the sedative lavenders could be detected on the breath, just moments after application to the skin. Or that the aromatic messenger and CNS-stimulant, cineole, would enable a rat to better negotiate a maze, whether it be inhaled, ingested or topically applied. And who would have guessed that Rosemary, the herb of Remembrance, would prove to contain nearly a dozen different aromatic compounds which slow the breakdown of acetylcholine, the mental messenger molecule often deficient in individuals with Alzheimer's and senile dementia. Who among us can describe the aroma that tells us that Cherry Birch and Wintergreen in the North Woods, and the Polygala in the South Woods share the same chemical, that pleasant anodyne, methyl salicylate? Who would not be surprised by the identical aromas of Chile's Boldo (*Peumus boldus*) and Maryland's Epazote (*Chenopodium ambrosioides*), a completely unrelated species, except chemically? Soon, the sniffer realizes that they both contain ascaridole, a useful compound, but dangerous, like all chemicals, natural and synthetic because in overdoses it upsets the body's homeostatic chemical reactions. Who can describe the unique aroma of the Sweet Annie, alias qinghao (*Artemisia annua*) unlike any other plant, unlike even any of the 500 Artemisias. We identify it by its odor, but cannot describe it, since it is unlike any other. It is not at all like the moxa or mugwort, *Artemisia vulgaris* being burned at the Santa Cruz Herbal Rebirthing. It smells so much like burning grass that some Native Americans and Chinese acupuncturists have been arrested on marijuana charges. JAMA's Armistice Day issue in 1998 reported clinical studies showing that moxibustion with *Artemisia vulgaris* could lower the incidence of breech births in the first pregnancy.

The modern acceptance of ancient plant knowledge has opened the minds and eyes of many converts. Despite this, many are walking around blind. The information superhighway is full of sound bites, but nothing of real sustenance. What do the names mean, what are the differences in where the plant is grown and what part is used and how does it work? Most of us never consider these details. Why not? When you meet a new person, don't you want to find out where they are from, what their life experience has been, what they like and don't like? Unless you ask, how do you really get to know them and without these details, what will set them apart from the other faces in the crowd?

*375 Essential Oils and Hydrosols* is the aromatic equivalent of an introduction service. Let Jeanne Rose do the 'scentual' introductions. She has dug into closets and unearthed secrets. Her storehouse of information includes personal histories, family trees, with similarities and differences, individual do's and don'ts; likes and dislikes, and personal stories to make the plants come alive.

Jeanne Rose does it again, detailing the aromatic world in a new light. In this book she combines ancient and the modern biochemical knowledge, along with her revolutionary experiences, and decades of hands-on involvement in aroma and body products, natural cosmetics and medicines, these are the 'naturals' for which Americans are increasingly clamoring. Laid out for the reader in thoughtful detail are the secrets, essences, and aromatic molecules of some of our most fragrant friends, presented to you by The Grand Dame of Aromatic and Cosmetic Herbals.

—James A. "Jim" Duke, Ph.D.
Former ethnobotanist, USDA
Director, Duke's Herbal Vineyard
Fulton, Maryland, Fall, 1998

# Introduction

If it is true that the word *aromathérapie* was coined by the French chemist René-Maurice Gattefossé in the 1930s and that medical aromatherapy is known and applied by thousands of French doctors and their colleagues pharmacists, it is similarly true that we attend in the North American Continent and especially in the USA, to an exponential growth of the use of essential oils. This authentic 'Aromatic Revolution,' the fourth one on planet Earth, entails, in a country full of contrasts like the US, 'the worst and the best.'

Some individuals become 'certified aromatherapists' after a few days of training and many books are mere 'copies of copies of copies'...with all the mistakes and inaccuracies involved by a hasty work of compilation!

Fortunately, this new book by Jeanne Rose belongs to the category of 'the best' and it is a delight for me to introduce the reader to the modestly entitled *375 Essential Oils and Hydrosols* whose reading gave me such pleasure and a inspiring global perspective. As Jeanne Rose points out clearly:

> *I view aromatherapy as a branch of herbalism,*
> *and learning when use of the herb is preferable*
> *to use of the essential oil is an important*
> *aspect of aromatherapy training.*

Thanks to her encompassing understanding of the vegetal kingdom and its uncountable and powerful resources, Jeanne Rose takes the reader in a travel that remains always refreshing and exciting, rich in personal reflections and live experience, be it on herself or with her students or clients.

I have been involved with natural medicine for over thirty years and I have practiced extensively and intensively medical aromatherapy for over twenty years. My first 'blessing' was to be introduced to the molecular understanding of EOs through my initiation with Pierre Franchomme. This is a necessary analytical stage that needs to be assimilated; it needs also to be integrated into a larger frame of reference, more holistically oriented. My second blessing was to perceive the reality and subtlety of the approach developed by English style aromatherapists. The third blessing was to be inspired in order to conceive a frame of thinking and working that I call 'Integral Aromatherapy,' where the Yang, scientifically oriented French style concept is perfectly complemented by the Yin, intuitive inspired English style way of perceiving and practicing.

In the teaching and in the work of Jeanne Rose, I can feel and recognize the existence of both influences, each at their own place, without any conflict about which one is superior to the other! In fact, the only 'superiority' lies in their conjunction and their unification, in the same way as a human being need his/her intellectual left brain and her/his artistic right brain working in perfect harmony.

On the one hand, Jeanne Rose, over decades of learning the scientific and botanical side has trained her intellectual brain in the best possible way; this accounts for the clarity and the accuracy of her presentation. On the other hand, living almost in osmosis with the world of plants since her early childhood, her intuitive brain was in no way 'strangulated or stifled' by the intellectual counterpart. This is why I acknowledge in her work this integral approach to essential oil's which I find so fascinating and so promising for the integral medicine of the next century.

I enjoyed very much the taxonomical approach and the botanical description of the overall perspective of the aromatic vegetal kingdom, topics which are rarely exposed in current English aromatherapy books.

I was fascinated to learn many details about The Aromatic Plant Project and the production of high quality hydrosols from organically grown plants by US farmers. I can only say "Bravo" and let aromatic plants be grown and floral and herbal waters (hydrosols) be produced from Florida to Alaska, from Texas to Idaho and from

California to Labrador. I loved the chapter Essential Oils Are More Than Stinky and all that Jeanne Rose wrote about the complete sensory experience. In itself, Chapter 3 is a pure jewel of reading and doing.

And I was thrilled to discover that the right time for conifers EOs to begin to be recognized for their incredible power is coming with Jeanne Rose's book. It is already a very significant step to devote a full chapter to the Conifers, who are so often confused and left on the side in most other aromatherapy books. This first accurate description of the aromatic initiators on planet Earth is to my eyes auspicious for the advent of their full recognition in the close future, when my work entitled "The First Aromatic Revolution and the World of the Conifers" will be translated and published in English.

When I discovered that Jeanne Rose had received the inspiration of including this Conifers chapter, it was for me the absolute confirmation that we are on similar wavelengths and that we share 'above spirit guides' that help us increasing the collective aromatic awareness which symbolizes the Fourth Aromatic Revolution we live nowadays all over the planet.

I am convinced that this comprehensive book will prove quite helpful both for 'old aromatherapists' who will brush up their knowledge and for newly trained aromatherapists who will be at once on a serious track that they will from then on follow with earnestness and passion.

Jeanne Rose, who is accomplished in reading French, played a major role in creating the French-American connection with her involvement in the first and original translation into English of Gattefossé's book.

This new guide represents a step further on the road that leads us towards better understanding, respect, and acceptance, and finally to a harmonious cooperation between all of us engaged in this planetary salvation task.

I wholeheartedly thank Jeanne Rose for her precious contribution. I know we will have a lot to share in the coming years.

—Daniel Pénoël, M.D.
Drôme Valley, December, 1998

# Introduction to the Author

I first read Jeanne Rose's *Herbs and Things* in 1972 while living on a houseboat moored at Gate 6 on Sausalito's colorful waterfront. The word aromatherapy was not yet used at that time in the United States, but as I read about the properties of essential oils that she mentioned, the seed of curiosity was planted in my mind. Over the past ten years I have had the good fortune to get to know her better.

Jeanne Rose is a medical herbalist, educator, author and president emeritus of the National Association for Holistic Aromatherapy (NAHA). With degrees in zoology and marine biology, as well as graduate research in herbs and pesticides, she combines an academic discipline with her hands-on knowledge of healing plants. I would like to give my impression of the scent of this remarkable woman, the essence of Jeanne Rose.

She embodies what the Welsh poet Dylan Thomas called "the force that through the green fuse drives the flower." And she is a force of nature, a presence to be reckoned with. She is a dynamic and dedicated visionary activist who gets her hands dirty with the experience of growing, harvesting, and distilling aromatic plants. She radiates a discerning sense of holistic wisdom as she pollinates her students with a knowledge of plant identification, botany, chemistry, and practical usage.

Jeanne's own garden at her Carl Street home in San Francisco is planted with a great variety of herbs and flowers, including her legendary Lemon Verbena tree. In her workshops, she shares her passion for distilling essential oils and especially hydrosols—the aromatic waters which have a wide range of uses including health, beauty and skin care.

Thinking of the big picture, Jeanne Rose initiated The Aromatic Plant Project (APP) in 1990. The mission of the APP is to encourage a grass roots movement of small scale local growers and distillers who plant and distill quality therapeutic aromatic plants, and consumers, who use these products. The aim is to evolve a sustainable agriculture of a variety of aromatic crops which produce exceptional essential oils and hydrosols. The resulting crop diversification and distillation is the way of the future, proclaiming that variety is truly the spice of life.

Every time that I hear her talk about the APP at conferences, I feel her animated enthusiasm for the project. Distillation is envisioned as a combined art and craft with obvious parallels to vintage wine making. Central to this theme is the concept of terroir—the ecological atmosphere of a location which influences the aromatic composition of plants—the sum of the terrain, soil, water, light, shade, wind, plus other flora and fauna. In geomancy, we refer to this as "the spirit of place." Terroir is the essence of holistic systems thinking.

Jeanne's *375 Essential Oils and Hydrosols* is a synesthetic invitation to experience the joys of aromatic plants. Similar to a wine appreciation guide, she describes scent types, the taste, viscosity, and the colors evoked by the imagination on sampling an essence.

Many of her students know the therapeutic, behavioral, skin care, and perfume uses of essential oils, but cannot recognize the plants from which these essences originate. Jeanne Rose ceaselessly campaigns to rectify this botanical illiteracy under the banner of the APP. And she has generously bequeathed her rare and extensive herbal library to the distinguished Lloyd Library in Cincinnati, Ohio, and her collection of herb medicine bottles and botanical prints to the American Botanical Council in Austin, Texas.

As a botanical ambassador she spreads the aromatic word far and wide, educating consumers to the beneficial uses of essential oils and hydrosols. Her teaching schedule in her "AROMAtherapy 2037" newsletter, which includes aromatherapy classes in Jamaica, Martha's Vineyard, Texas, and British Columbia, reads like ads in a travel magazine. She does not let moss grow under her feet.

Jeanne is a Green Woman who embodies committed aromatic action. There she goes in her Honda stuffed with 250 pounds of lavender just harvested in Santa Barbara on a mad relay drive with her son, the lavender to be distilled in Sonoma, she trails fragrant clouds of glory down the California highways.

—John Steele, Aromatic Consultant
Sherman Oaks, California, December 1998

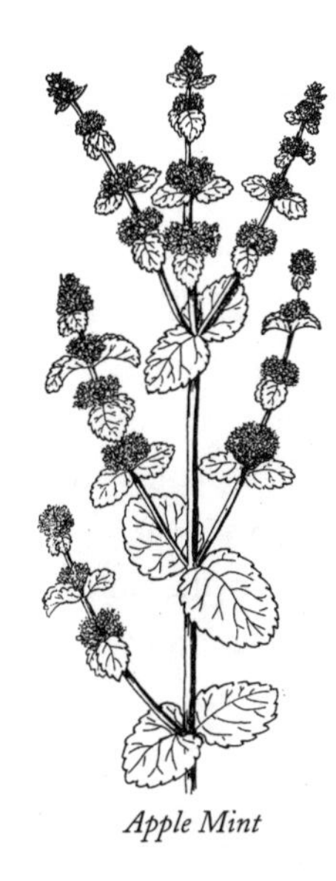

*Apple Mint*

ONE

# Introduction to Aromatherapy Botany

## Why Botany?

It's good to know basic plant structure or morphology, which comes from the Greek word *morphos*, meaning form. Learning botany is in some ways like learning a new language, difficult, but, definitely worthwhile. Once one understands the language and begins to become aware of the terms of their meaning, it allows for a sharpening of one's focus and ability to differentiate between plant families and different types of plants. The advantage of learning terms is that it organizes one's perception, so that one can actually see patterns in the plant world.[1]

Knowledge of these botanical patterns, in combination with intuition, helps hone the skills of the practicing aromatherapist in choosing oils to match clients' patterns in order to create the perfect fit of health and beauty; furthermore, a clear understanding of botany will afford the aromatherapist a more precise and broad ranging ability in developing synergistic blends. As research projects and scientific papers in aromatherapy grow, this knowledge will be essential.

[1]Inspired by H. J. Fuller and O. Tippo, *College Botany* (New York: Henry Holt, 1948).

## Why Taxonomy?

Taxonomy is the study of plant classification and relationships. It's also called *systematic botany*. It's needed because there are so many kinds of plants; at least 500,000 living species have been described. A top taxonomist may only be able to identify 5000 species.

There are several systems of classification. Pliny, A.D. 23–79, used size and form as criteria and established three primary groupings—herbs, shrubs, and trees. During the Middle Ages plants were described on the basis on their use: medicinal plants, edible plants, and poisonous plants. Linnaeus (Carolus Linnaeus, a great Swedish botanist, 1707–1778) established a classification based on the number of stamens. Stamens were considered to be sex organs, and many of Linnaeus' contemporaries considered his system to be obscene. These three systems are considered *artificial systems*: they consist of classes set up arbitrarily.

A *natural system*, on the other hand, is based on natural relationships. In other words, similar plants are placed in groups based on their true affinities to one another. Typically, the simpler plants are placed first, and the more complex ones follow. Essentially, natural systems reflect evolution. Natural systems of classification are relatively recent in origin. Their development is based upon the accumulated research and interpretation of structure and development of generations of botanists.

## Definition of Terms

*Genus* (Latin for race or kind)—a group of closely related species. The first part of the Latin binomial (e.g. *Artemisia*) is the name of the plant. Its first letter is always capitalized, and it is written in italics.

*Species* (sp=a specie) (spp=species) (L. species–form, kind)—usually the smallest unit in the classification of organisms; a group of individuals of the same ancestry, of nearly identical structure and behavior, and of relative stability in nature. The individuals of a species ordinarily interbreed freely and maintain themselves and their characteristics in nature. The second part of the Latin binomial name is written in lower case (e.g. *Artemisia arborescens*), and it is written in italics.

*Subspecies* (ssp=subspecies)—subdivision of a species; a taxonomic category that generally is the lowest used below a species, designating a *morphologically* distinguishable group whose members are at least partially or wholly *isolated* geographically. Think of such plants and animals as those of the Galapagos Islands (e.g. *Citrus aurantium* ssp. aurantium).

*Variety/subspecies (var/ssp)*—often a named, cloned type. (Think of wine, such as the 200 varieties of Cabernet). It is an inferior category to a species, and has nothing to do with geographical isolation.

*Variety*—Like the subspecies, the variety has been employed in several ways. It is often used today for local facies (the particular look) of species (apparently comprising a few biotypes), morphologically distinct and occupying a restricted geographical area (DuRietz, 1930; Rothmaler, 1994). Emphasis is on the small-scale, more localized range of the variety, compared with the large-scale, regional basis of the subspecies (Heywood, 1959a). In this sense, varieties may be geographical, ecological (ecotypes), cytological (cytodemes), or a combination of these (several varieties are often recognized within one subspecies). The variety is also used for variations whose precise nature is not understood; a treatment often necessary in the pioneer phase of taxonomy.

This distributional hierarchical construction is to some extent independent of the morphological differences involved: subspecies may differ from one another in fewer and less well-marked characters than varieties or even forms within the same species.

*Race*—an intraspecific category characterized by conspicuous physiological (physiological race), biological (biological race), geographical (geographical race), or ecological (ecological race) properties. Usually restricted to animal groupings (e.g. in humans: Asian, Caucasian, etc.).

*Breed*—usually reserved for animals. A group of organisms related by descent; an artificial mating group having a common ancestor; used specifically in genetic studies of domesticated species (e.g., for cows: Angus, Hereford, Guernsey, Holstein).

*Cultivated Variety (CV)*—made and cultivated by man, also called a Cultivar–not made by nature. (e.g., in Lavender, *Lavandula* x *intermedia* cv: Abriali, Super, Grosso)

*Clone*—propagation of a particular plant by budding or by cuttings through many vegetative generations (nonsexual).

*Chemotype (CT)*—chemical composition of the essential oil where one chemical dominates over the norm–is dependent on terroir (e.g., in Basil, *Ocimum basilicum* CT, Linaloöl, thymol, eugenol, etc.)

## Terroir

A French word that reflects the expression of the earth, the particular planting site (its topology), in the resultant essential oil. The factors of soil, shade, wind, water, altitude, rain, and terrain make up the terroir.

One of the mystiques of essential oils is the variations available. First, let's consider some of the variables in agriculture.

*Clone Type* (Clonal selection of the variety)—Clones are like identical twins but even closer, yet they show some different characteristics that can have a rather dramatic difference in the end product. As an example, there are over twenty-five different identified clonal selections of Basil.

*Where Planted* (Location of the planting)—Any place, while only a relatively small area in relation to other growing regions of the world, exhibits widely different soil types, depths, textures, drainage, fertility, slopes (from steep hillsides to flat land), sun exposure, altitude, etc. Even within a small property, we see finite differences within a small distance.

*Weather* (Weather variations)—The amount of rainfall and the time of year in which it falls can directly affect flower and seed size, chemical concentration,and health of the plant. We see a wide variation of rainfall within any area. Regarding local temperature, there are hot spots and cool spots in any area.

*Location* (Location relative to the water or mountains and the amount of wind present are also factors)—Finally, there are the year-to-year weather variations, which can be significant. In recent years there have been both unusually hot seasons and long, cool growing seasons.

A significant number of variables have been covered here without even touching on growing or distillation techniques, which are some of the most important variables. We will talk about these later.

## Why Do Plants Smell?

We read in *Leaflet* magazine that plants have a scent for two basic reasons: *defense* and *attraction.* The essential oil smell from leaf, root, and bark **defend** plants against being browsed or chewed; flower and fruit scents **attract** animals for pollination and seed dispersal. The goals of these two strategies are often diametrically opposed. For example, the Western Azalea (*Rhododendron occidentale*) has skunk scented leaves but the flowers are sweetly perfumed.

Leaves are often covered with a mass of tiny cells filled with smelly molecules known as volatile, essential, or ethereal oils. Many of these oils belong chemically to a family of compounds called terpenes. Not only do these oils render the leaves unappetizing or downright sickening to animals seeking a meal, they also evaporate readily on hot days to cool the leaf surfaces. In addition, some of these terpenes have been implicated with inhibiting the growth of neighboring plants and seeds when they are carried into the soil on water droplets.

Flower fragrances are primary or secondary attractants of pollinators. Pollinators may be attracted to flowers from a distance by a combination of color, shape, and fragrance, although all of these factors may not be involved for all pollinators. For example, dung beetles are strongly attracted to certain aromas such as the putrid odor of the spadix of the Voodoo Lily (*Sauromatum guttatum*). The putrid odor is caused when certain amine-containing molecules are broadcast efficiently and far as the flowers' spadix heats up. Many tropical bats are attracted by the odor of overripe fruit. Hawkmoths hone in on flowers from some distance when they perceive the cloyingly sweet odors of such night bloomers as Angel's Trumpet (*Datura* spp.), night-blooming Jasmine (*Cestrum noctiflorum)*, and Nicotianas (*Nicotiana* sp.).

Other flowers offer scent that is only perceptible at short range, and sometimes only when the pollinator has already landed on the flower. By providing cues in the form of color guides and odor trails, these flowers help guide pollinators to their reward of pollen or nectar. Many members of the pea family (Fabaceae) and orchid family (Orchidaceae) are particularly noted for their specific odor patterns.

The nature of flower odors varies according to the group of pollinators that are attracted: Flowers that attract bees and butterflies often have pleasantly sweet fragrances but not necessarily overpowering ones. Flowers that attract moths are typified by heavily cloying, sweet odors. Flowers attractive to bats often produce musky or rotting fruit odors. Flowers attractive to dung beetles and flys have—at least to humans—spectacularly unpleasant odors, typified by the names of the compounds involved: putracine, skatol, and cadaverine.

The strength of the scent of plants is also a factor of terroir. Terroir is a factor of soil, shade, water, altitude, rain, and terrain.

## How Plants Store Essential Oils

Aromatic substances are formed and stored in certain organs of a plant as by-products or as the end result of its metabolism.

*Glandular Cells, Glandular Hairs, and Glandular Scales*—These are single or multi-cell protuberances, or 'pockets,' on the surface of the plant's epidermis. Plants that store essential oils in this manner include: Thyme, Marjoram, Rosemary, Sage (that is, all of the family Lamiaceae [Labiates]).

*Oil Cells and Resin Cells*—These are cells (still living in some cases) which are filled with oil or resin in plants of the Laurel family (Lauraceae). These include Laurel leaves, Cinnamon, and Cassia.

*Oil or Resin Canals*—Inter-cellular spaces in plant tissues store essential oils and resin. When adjoining glandular cells move apart, the spaces expand into tubular canals or ducts. Essential oils formed in this way are found in the schizocarp fruits of the Apiaceae (Umbellifers). These include Caraway, Aniseed, Fennel, Coriander, and Celery.

Conifers, too, have resin canals. Large quantities of resin can be extracted from a damaged tree. Some resins are gathered by the method of 'tapping.'

*Oil Reservoirs*—Lysigenous secretory reservoirs are formed inside a plant as the wall. Secretory cells gradually disintegrate. This is called secondary cavity formation. Particularly noted for their lysigenous cavities, or oil reservoirs are the Rue family (Rutaceae) and Citrus varieties, including Lemon, Orange, and Bergamot.

Kurt Schnaubelt, writing in his book *Medical Aromatherapy*, has made some interesting comments regarding standards in essential oils. "Essential oils may be impossible to standardize because they reflect the intrinsic variability of nature…essential oils should be as rich and complex as they are when they come out of the still. Seasonal or yearly variations (or variations originating from different distillation processes) should be permitted because they are the legitimate expression of the regional geographic and climatic influences as well as the interaction of the grower with nature in crafting the oil."

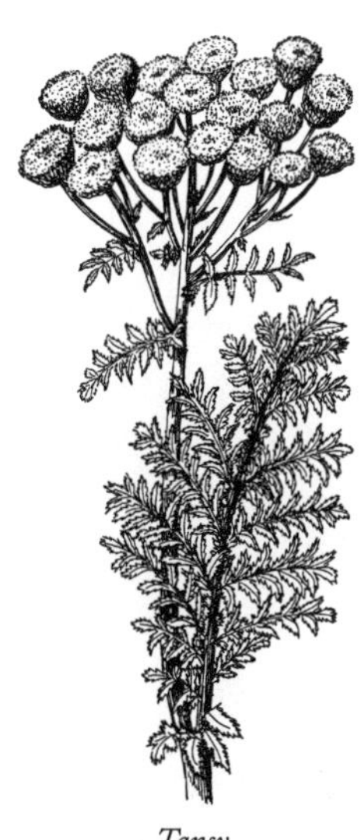

*Tansy*

# TWO

# Plant Names Mean Something

When plants are named, botanists classify them according to their relationship to other plants. Their individual names are often given to describe an attribute of the plant. In these common and technical names you can find a history of botany, a romance of adventure, and for the adventurous it can be a mental trip to far lands and ancient worlds. Found here are descriptions of natural habitats, colors, and scent which are described and noted. With this new vocabulary, you will be better able to determine where a plant was originally found, who found it, and where you might go to look for it in a natural environment. Knowing the name of something and what it means will provide useful clues and tools to aid you in your plant research.

I will linguistically dissect as many plant names as I know. Some definitely need more research and I urge you to obtain two books: *The Plant Book* by D. J. Mabberly and *Jaeger's Source Book of Biological Names and Terms* by Edmund C. Jaeger. *The Plant Book* is a dictionary of the higher plants, including common names, Latin binomials, who named the plant, family name, and habitat. *Jaeger's Source Book of Biological Names and Terms* defines the terms simply, while giving some background; I have had my copy since I attended San Jose State College in 1956. It has served me well all these years, and I still take pleasure in reading it. Jaeger dedicated this book to David Starr Jorden, "who had the good sense, when coining generic names, to explain their origin so that those who followed him could have no doubt concerning their exact connotation. He was seldom, if ever, given to the making of so-called nonsense names for he saw in every well-made scientific name a treasure house of meaning carrying valuable clues to identification, rich allusions to scientific history and discovery."

You might also wish to befriend the fantastic librarian at the Helen Crocker Russel Library in Strybing Arboretum in Golden Gate Park, San Francisco, CA.; Barbara Pitschel who enjoys the hunt and detective work of chasing down obscure adventurous names of plants.

**Allspice (*Pimenta officinalis*)**
*Pimenta* = pepper; *officinalis* = used officially

**Ambretta (*Hibiscus abelmoschus, H. moschatus*)**
*Hibiscus* = the marsh mallow; *abelmoschus* = from the Arabic, father of musk (refers to the musk-scented seeds); *moscheutes* = musk-scented

***Ammi visnaga***
*Ammi* = an African plant; *visnaga* = toothpick

***Amyris balsamifera***
*Amyris* = Balsam; *balanifera* = bearing acornlike parts

**Angelica (*Angelica archangelica*)**
*Angelica* = angelic medicinal properties; *archangelica* = archangel Raphael

**Anise seed (*Pimpinella anisum*)**
*Pimpinella* = pimpernel; *anisum* = anise

***Artemisia arborescens***
*Artemisia* = after the Goddess Artemis; *arborescens* = becoming treelike

***Artemisia douglasiana***
*Artemisia* = after the Goddess Artemis; *douglasiana* = after David Douglas (1798–1834), a Scottish botanist killed in Hawaii by the native Hawaiians. He made several scientific journeys to the Americas, spending most of his time in California and collecting for the Horticultural Society of London

**Balsam Peru (*Myroxylon pereirae*)**
*Myro* = sweet oil or perfume; *xylon* = wood; *balsamum* = balsum; *pereirae* = from the port of Peru.

Myroxylon balsamum var. pereirae derives its name from Callao, Peru, the port of export, although the center of commercial production lay in northwestern El Salvador.

According to Lloyd, "The substance was mentioned in all the early editions (of the *USP*) under the name *Myroxylon* until 1850, when the modern name [*Balsamum Peruvianum] was employed.* In consequence of the fact that the exports of Guatemala came through the port of Lima, Peru. The misleading name of "Peruvian Balsam" was in the early days affixed to it, paralleling somewhat the record of "Mocha Coffee," which is not grown in Mocha, or even thereabouts, but was exported therefrom in the early days of Arabian coffee."

**Balsam Tolu (*Toluifera balsamum, Myroxylon balsamum, Myrosperum toluiferum*)**

*Toluifera* = Tolu balsam, first brought from Santiago de Tolu, a seaport of Columbia; *balsamum* = balsam

**Sweet Basil (*Ocimum basilicum*)**

*Ocimum* = a sort of clover or aromatic plant; *basilicum* = comes from the Greek word meaning a petty king, royal, princely, or a kind of serpent with a spot on its head like a crown.

**Bay (*Laurus nobilus*)**

*Laurus* = evergreen trees, Laurel; *nobilus* = notable, or noble, or noble.

**Bay Rum (*Pimenta racemosa*)**

*Pimenta* = pepper; *racemosa* = prone to producing a cluster of berries

**Benzoin (*Styrax benzoin*)**

*Styrax* = an ancient name for a tree producing a fragrant gummy resin called "storax" by Pliny, can also mean the spike at the lower end of a spear shaft; *benzoin* = the frankincense of Java

**Bergamot (*Citrus bergamia*)**

*Citrus* = like a citrus; *bergamia* = after an Italian town where the tree was first observed

**Birch Bark (*Betula lenta*)**

*Betula* = the birch; *lenta* = tough, but flexible

**Birch Tar (*Betula spp.*) (i.e., *pubescens, alba, pendula*)**

*Betula* = the birch; *pubescens* = refers to the downy hairs of puberty; *alba* = white; *pendula* = pendulous branchlets

**Black Pepper (*Piper nigrum*)**

*Piper* = pepper; *nigrum* = dark or black

**Bois de Rose oil (*Aniba rosaeodora*)**

*Aniba* = a Tupi Indian name; *rosaeodora* = fragrance like a rose

**Borneol (*Dryobalanops aromatica*)**

*Dryobalanops* = *dryo,* which means tree, *balan,* which means acorn or male glans and *ops*, which means appearing like; *aromatica* = aromatic

**Cabreuva (*Myocarpis frondosus*)**

*Myocarpis* = from the Greek word *myron* which means sweet oil or perfume and *karpos* meaning the fruit. Myocarpis means a sweet perfumed fruit or the sweet product from the fruit; *frondosus* = full of leaves

**Cade (*Juniperis oxycedrus*)**

*Juniperis* = like a evergreen, conifer, or juniper; *oxycedrus* = sharply pointed leaves like a cedar, unlike a juniper. Also, oxy can refer to cedar which loves acid soil.

**Cajeput oil (*Melaleuca minor, M. leucadendron*)**

*Melaleuca* = from *mela* which means black and *leuca* which means white, referring to the description of the contrasting black and white colors of the peeling bark; *minor* = small

***Calamintha nepeta* ssp. *nepeta***

*Calamintha* = beautiful mint, *nepeta* ssp. *nepeta* = scorpion, which is a name used by Pliny, or a related genus; *nepeta* = from Latin for catnip and from Nepi, Italy.

**Calamus (*Acorus calamus*)**

*Acorus* = sweet-flag; *calamus* = reedlike

**Calendula (*Calendula officinalis*)**

*Calendula* = refers to the the first day of the month or the calends, which refers to the long flowering period; *officinalis* = a plant used officially in medicine

***Calophyllum inophyllum* (Kamani Tree)**

*Calo* = beautiful; *inophyllum* = *ino* which could refer to a sea goddess or a fiber, and *phyllum* which means leaves

**Camomile**

**Roman Chamomile (*Chamæmelum nobile*)**

*Chamæmelum*= *chamae* which means to be on the ground, low-growing, or dwarflike, and *mel* which means smells like honey; *nobile* = noble

German or Hungarian Chamomile (***Matricaria recutita***)

*Matricaria* = refers to the womb or often used in the sense of a place where something is generated; *recutita* = having a fresh or new skin, also circumcised

**Moroccan Chamomile** or **Ormenis mixta** (***Chamaemelum mixtum***)

*Chamaemelum* = from *chamae* which means to be on the ground or dwarflike and *mel* which means smells like honey; *mixtum* = looks like both plants mixed together

**Camphor** (***Cinnamomum camphora***)

*Cinnamomum* = cinnamon; *camphora* = camphorlike

**Cananga** (***Cananga odorata***)

*Cananga* = flower of flowers; *odorata* = sweet smelling

**Caraway** (***Carum carvi***)

*Carum* = Greek name of caraway; *carvi* = Latin name for caraway

**Carrot Seed** (***Daucus carota***)

*Daucus* = name of an umbelliferous plant; *carota* = from the Greek word for carrot

**Cassia bark** (***Cinnamomum cassia***)

*Cinnamomum* = cinnamon; *cassia* = an ancient name for some leguminous plants, some relate this to *cantha*, which means thorns or to the Acacia.

**Cedar** (often used improperly for trees of two different families, Pinaceae and Cupressaceae)

**Cedarleaf** or **Thuja** (***Thuja occidentalis***)

*Thuja* = from the Greek name of a juniper or meaning African tree with fragrant, durable wood or meaning the arbor vitae or Tree of Life; *occidentalis* = means westerly or west

**Cedarwood "Atlas"** (***Cedrus atlantica***)

*Cedrus* = true cedar or resinous tree; *atlantica* = of the Atlantic and the Atlas Mountains and refers to Atlas, the gigantic God who bore up the pillers of Heaven

**Cedarwood, East African** (***Juniperus procera***)

*Juniperus* = juniper; *procera* = means stretched out, prostrate

**Himalaya Cedarwood** (***Cedrus deodora***)

*Cedrus* = true cedar or resinous tree; *deodora* = an Indian word for 'the divine tree,' or Tree of the Gods

**Lebanon Cedar (*Cedrus libani*)**

*Cedrus* = true cedar or resinous tree; *libani* = refers to the plant from Mount Lebanon

**Port Orford Cedarwood (*Chamæcyparis lawsoniana*)**

*Chamæcyparis* = a low-growing cypress; *lawsoniana* = named after Charles Lawson (1794–1874), Edinburgh nurseryman who raised the tree from its original introduction in 1854, it is called the Lawson Cypress

**Texas Cedarwood (*Juniperus mexicana*)**

*Juniperus mexicana* = the juniper from Mexico

**Chilé (Red) Pepper (*Capsicum annuum*)**

*Capsicum* = to bite, referring to the hot taste; *annuum* = annual

**Cinnamon (*Cinnamomum zeylanicum*)**

*Cinnamomum* = cinnamon; *zeylanicum* = Ceylon

**Citron (*Citrus medica*)**

*Citrus* = citrus; *medica* = healing or curative

**Citronella (*Cymbopogon nardus*)**

*Cymbopogon* = from *cymba* which means from the Latin cymbo or boat, and *pogon* which means bearded or the shape of the bracts, meaning the racemes are enclosed by bracts that resemble spathes; *nardus* = nard, an Indian or Assyrian plant yielding a fragrant substance for unguents

**Citrus Scents** Citrus means citrus

*Citrus aurantium* = orange colored

*Citrus bergamia* = means Bergamot, after the Italian town

*Citrus limonum* peel

*limonum*=a bright or flowery surface or meadow, name for lemon

*Citrus medica* = healing or curative, used in medicine

*Citrus nobilis* = noble

*Citrus paradisi* = paradise or a pleasure ground

*Citrus reticulata* peel

*reticulata* = made like a net

*Citrus vulgaris* = common

**Clary Sage (*Salvia sclarea*)**

*Salvia* = whole or sound, refers to the sap or the medicinal properties; *sclarea* = refers to the sclera or white of the eyeball and here refers to the seeds and leaves used to clear obstruction in the eye

**Cloves (*Syzygium aromatica*)**
*Syzygium* = a joining or yoking together; *aromatica* = aromatic

**Clove bark (*Dicypellium caryophyllatum*)**
*Dicypellium* = *di* which means two and *cypellium* is from the Greek, *Kypellon* or a beaker, cup or goblet; *caryophyllatum* = clove-leaved, a kind of plant, the clove tree

**Copaiba (*Copaifera officinalis*)**
*Copaifera* could come from a report from Petrus Martys to Pope Leo X referring to a South American tree called copei, which meant plentiful, or a South American river called Copaibo; *officinalis* = used officially in medicine

**Coriander (*Coriandrum sativum*)**
*Coriandrum* = an ancient name for coriander; *sativum* = that which is sown or grown

**Croton (*Croton eluteria*)**[Other common name = ***Cascarilla* bark**]
*Croton* = a tick or a bug; *eluteria* = to wash off

**Cubeb (*Piper cubeba*)**
*Piper* = pepper; *cubeba* = cubeb

**Cumin (*Cuminum cyminum*)**
*Cuminum* = an aromatic herb; *cyminum* = cumin seed)

**Cyclamen (*Cyclamen europaeum*)**
*Cyclamen* = Greek name for cornous herbs, sow bread; *europaeum* = from Europe

**Cypress (*Cupressus sempervirens*)** several trees are termed Cypress including Cupressus and Chamaecyparis and others
*Cupressus* = the cypress; *sempervirens* = always green

**Dill Seed or Weed(*Anethum graveolens*)**
*Anethum* = dill or anise; *graveolens* = heavily scented

**Douglas Fir (*Pseudotsuga menziesii*)**
*Pseudotsuga* = false larch or false evergreen conifer; *menziesii* = named after Archibald Menzies (1754–1842), naval surgeon and naturalist to Vancouver's Pacific coast expedition. This is the same plant that is also called *Pseudotsuga douglasii.*

**Elemi (*Canarium commune*)**
*Canarium* = from a Malai word meaning the Java almond; *commune* = common

**Eucalyptus** (***Eucalyptus spp.***)

*Eucalyptus* = well covered, referring to the calyx which forms a lid over the flowers in bud

*E. globulus* = like a globe

*E. australiana* = from Australia

*E. radiata* = spoke-like, radiating

*E. citriodora* = smells like lemon

*E. campanulata* = bellshaped

**Fennel** (***Fœniculum vulgare***)

*Fœniculum* = haylike; *vulgare* = common

**Fir Needle** includes ***Abies, Larix, Abies sibirica*** or ***Abies balsamea***

*Abies* = the classical name for Firs; *alba* = white and refers to the bark of old trees; *balsamea* = meaning balsam producing, referring to the bark

**Frankincense** (***Boswellia carterii***)

*Frankincense* = the true or real incense; *Boswellia* = an important genus of incense-bearing trees, named after James Boswell; *carterii* = after Professor Carter who described the Egyptian mummies

**Galanga** (***Alpina officinarum***)

*Alpina* = alpine; *officinarum* = refers to its nature or use

**Galbanum** (***Ferula galbanifera***)

*Ferula* = fennel; *galbanifera* = the greenish-yellow resin of certain plants of Syria

**Garlic oil** (***Allium sativum***)

*Allium* = garlic; *sativum* = that which is sown

**Geranium, Rose Geranium, African** or **Algerian Geranium** (***Pelargonium graveolens*** or ***Pelargonium asperum***)

*Pelargonium* =from *pelargos* which means a stork and *gonium* referring to the shape of the bill of a stork and to the look of the flower parts of the plant, *graveolens*= heavily scented;

*asperum* = an uneven or rough place

**Ginger** (***Zingiber officinale***)

*Zingiber* = ginger of ancient orgin, probably pre-Roman, *srnga* which means a horn and *ver* which means a root; *officinale* = a plant officially used in medicine

**Gotu Kola** or **Indian Pennywort** (***Centella asiatica***)

*Centella* = to prick or puncture; *asiatica* = from Asia

**Grapefruit oil, Grapefruit seed oil** (*Citrus x paradisi* = the Citrus from Paradise)

***Helichrysum italicum***

*Helichrysum* = from *heli* which means the sun and *chrysum* which refers to the gold colors of the flowers; *italicum* = from Italy

**Heliotrope** (***Heliotropium peruvianum***)

***Heliotropium*** = from *Helio* meaning the sun and *tropium* which means to turn toward the sun; *peruvianum* = from Peru

**Honeysuckle** (***Lonicera caprifolium***)

*Lonicera* = after Adam Lonitzer (1528 - 1586), German naturalist; *caprifolium* from *capri*, meaning goat, and *folium*, meaning leaves

**Hinoki root** and **leaf** (***Chamaecyparis obtusa***)

*Chamaecyparis* = a low-growing cypress; *obtusa* = blunt or dull

**Hops** (***Humulus lupulus***)

*Humulus* = a version of an old German name or from the Latin humus, meaning soil and alluding to its "occasionally prostrate habit;" *lupulus* = a small wolf, from an old name, willow wolf, referring to its habit of climbing over willows

**Hyssop** (***Hyssopus officinalis***)

*Hyssopus* = an old name for another plant; *officinalis* = a plant officially used in medicine

**Inula** (***Inula graveolens*** or ***Inula odorata***)

*Inula* = the plant called elecampane; *graveolens* = heavily scented; *odorata* = odorous

**Iris** (***Iris spp.***)

*Iris* = refers to the rainbow

**Jasmine flower** (***Jasminum officinale*** and ***Jasminum grandiflorum***)

*Jasminum* = Arabic name for a particular shrub; *officinale* = officially used in medicine; *grandiflorum* = big flowers or a big inflorescence

**Juniper Berry** (***Juniperus communis*** )

*Juniperus* = juniper tree; *communis* = growing together

**Kewda** (***Pandanus odoratissimus***)

*Pandanus* = a Mali word meaning conspicious; *odoratissimus* = very fragrant

**Labdanum** (***Cistus ladanifer***)

*Cistus* = a flowering shrub, from a Greek word referring to a box or a capsule; *ladanifer* = from Portugal and refers to a gummy substance secreted by the plant

**Lanyana** (***Artemisia afra***)

*Artemisia* = refers to the Goddess Artemis; *afra* = Artemisia plant from Africa

**Lavender** (***Lavandula angustifolia*, *L. vera*** aka ***L. officinalis*** and ***L. latifolia***)

***Lavandula*** = refers to the word lavare = to wash, referring to the fact that it was used in laundry to make the clothes smell good; *angustifolia* = narrowleaved; *vera* = true; *officinalis* and *officinale* = means in common use or a plant officially used in medicine; *latifolia* = leaves on the side

**Lavandin** (***L. x intermedia cv Grosso, Abrialii***, etc.)

*intermedia* = in-between; *Grosso* = named by or after Mr. Grosso

**Lemon** (***Citrus limon***)

*limon* = citrus with a bright surface

**Lemon Mint** (***Mentha citrata***)

*citrata* = mint that smells like citrus

**Lemongrass** (***Cymbopogon citratus***)

*Cymbopogon*=from the Latin *cymbo* which means a boat, and *pogon*,which means bearded or the shape of the bracts, meaning the racemes are enclosed by bracts that resemble spathes; ***citratus*** = smells like citrus

**Lime** (***Citrus medica var. acida***)

*Citrus medica* = citrus that is curative

**Lovage herb, Lovage root** (***Levisticum officinale***)

*Levisticum* = refers to lovage used medicinally; *officinale* = plant officially used in medicine

**May Chang** (***Litsea cubeba***)

*Litsea* = a little plum; *cubeba* = the cubeb

**Mandarin** (***Citrus reticulata***)

*Citrus reticulata* = citrus with netlike membrane

**Marjoram** (***Origanum majorana***)

*Origanum* = refers to a plant that stretches and grows in all directions; *majorana* = the large form

**Mastic** (***Pistacia lentiscus***)

*Pistacia* = a type of tree, from Greek for pistachio nut; *lentiscus* = refers to mastic

**MQV** or **True Niaouli** (***Melaleuca quinquenervia viridiflora***)
*Melaleuca* = black and white contrast of the peeling bark on trunks and stems; *quinquenervia* = five parts; *viridiflora* = green flowers

**Melilot** (***Melilotus officinalis***)
*Melilotus* = honey-scented plant; *officinalis* = plant officially used in medicine

**Melissa** (***Melissa officinalis***)
*Melissa* = refers to the honeybee, because the plant attracts bees; *officinalis* = plant officially used in medicine

**Mimosa absolute** (***Acacia spp.***)
*Acacia* = means acacia and refers to a sharp point, the thorns

**Mint** (***Mentha arvensis***)
*Mentha arvensis* = mint that grows in a plowed field or a field weed

**Mugwort** (***Artemisia herba alba*** or ***A. vulgare***)
*Artemisia* = named for the ancient Goddess Artemis; *herba alba* = white herb; *vulgare* = common herb

**Myrrh** (***Commiphora molmol***, or ***C. myrrha***)
*Commiphora* = gumbearing; *molmol* = the original Somali word for this bitter, resinous exudation; *myrrha* = bitter

**Myrtle** (***Myrtus communis***)
*Myrtus* = the Greek and Latin name for the myrtle; *communis* = common

**Neroli** (***Citrus aurantium, C. vulgaris, C. bigaradia***)
*Citrus aurantium* = gold-colored citrus; *C. vulgaris* = common citrus; *C. bigaradia* =?

**Niaouli** (***Melaleuca viridiflora***) or **MQV**
*Melaleuca* = refers to the black and white contrast of the peeling bark on trunks and stems; *viridiflora* = green flowers

**Nutmeg** (***Myristica fragrans***)
*Myristica* = fit for anointing; *fragrans* = fragrant

**Oakmoss** (***Evernia prunastri***)
Oakmoss is not a moss, it is a lichen. *Evernia* = sprouts well; *prunastri* = *prun* which means prune or plum, and *astri*, which means sort of like, and may refer to the wrinkled look of the fruiting body

**Olibanum (*Boswellia carterii*)**

Olibanum = from an Arabic word *al luban* (the milk), referring to the appearance of the resin as it exudes from the tree; *Boswellia* = named for James Boswell (see frankincense); *carterii* = named after Professor Carter who studied mummies and opened tombs in Egypt where Olibanum was found

**Opopanax (*Commiphora erythraea*)**

*Commiphora* = gumbearing; *erythraea* = reddish

**Orange Flower**–See Neroli

**Orange Peel (*Citrus sinensis, C. aurantium dulcis*)**

*Citrus sinensis* = citrus from China; or *C. aurantium dulcis* = golden citrus that is sweet

**Oregano (*Origanum vulgare, Thymus capitatus*)**

*Origanum vulgare* = the common plant that spreads itself out; *Thymus* is Greek for soul=a word used for "to perfume, to sacrifice," perhaps because it was burned on altars; *capitatus* = having a head

**Orris (*Iris florentina* or *Iris pallida*)**

*Iris* = refers to the rainbow, because of the rainbow - colored flowers; *florentina* = the iris from Florence, refers to Flora, the Goddess of flowers; *pallida* = pale

**Oud** or **Aloes wood (*Aquileria malaccensis*)**

*Aquileria* = possibly from the Latin aquila, meaning eagle, or for the town of Aquileia in northern Italy; *malaccensis* = relates to Malacca on the Malay Peninsula

**Palmarosa (*Cymbopogon martinii*)**

Originally named by William Roxburgh (1751 - 1815) and revised by William Watson (1858–1925) after the *cymbopogon* = from *cymba*, which means from the Latin cymbo or boat, and *pogon*, which means bearded or the shape of the bracts, meaning the racemes are enclosed by bracts that resemble spathes; *Martinii*, common name Palmarosa, was named by William Roxberg (1751–1815). He was the Superintendent of the Calcutta Botanic Garden and Chief Botanist of the East India Company in 1793 to 1813. Roxberg states that this plant, "is plentiful in the Capital's Botanic Garden and was raised from seed that was sent me, from General Martin, who collected the seeds in the highlands of

Balla-ghat, while there with the army, during the last war with Tippoo Sultan. General Martin's name I have applied as a specific one for this elegant plant." General Martin sent Roxberg this grass from Lucknow and wrote, "I took particular notice of a sort of long grass which the cattle were voraciously fond of, which is of so strong an aromatic and pungent taste, that the flesh of the animals, as also the milk and butter, have a very strong scent of it. Of this grass I send you a small stalk, some roots, and seed; if you taste the latter, though old, you will find it of a very pungent aromatic taste."

**Parsley (*Petroselinum sativum*)**

*Petroselinum* = has to do with rocks; *sativum* = that which is sown

**Parsley Seed (*Petroselinum sativum*)**

**Patchouli (*Pogostemon patchouli*)**

*Pogostemon* = from *pogo,* which means bearded, and *stemon*, which means stamen of a flower; *patchouli* = patchouli

**Pennyroyal, American (*Hedeoma pulegioides*)**

*Hedeoma* = sweet smelling; *pulegioides* = has to do with fleas

**Pennyroyal, European (*Mentha pulegium*)**

*Mentha pulegium* = a pennyroyal mint

**Pepper (*Piper nigrum*)**

*Piper* = pepper; *nigrum* = black

**Pepper, California Pepper Tree (*Schinus molle*)**

*Schinus* = mastic plant; *molle* = the indigenous Peruvian name for this pepper tree, and refers to a word meaning soft

**Peppermint (*Mentha* x *piperita*)**

*Mentha* x *piperita* = pepper-scented mint

**Petitgrain (*Citrus aurantium*)**, sometimes called ***C. aurantium amara***

*Citrus aurantium* = golden citrus; *amara* = from the Greek word for trench, or the Latin for bitter, or the ancient Greek word meaning to shine

**Pine (*Pinus spp.*)**

*Pinus* = pine

***Ravensara anisata***

*Ravensara* = a Madagascar word; *anisata* = anise scented

***Ravensara aromatica***

*Ravensara* = a Madagascar word; *aromatica* = aromatic

**Rose**

*Rosa centifolia*

*Rosa* = rose; *centifolia* = 100 leafed

*Rosa damascena*

*Rosa* = rose; *damascena* = meaning from Damascus, Syria (Bulgaria)

*Rosa damascena bifera*

*Rosa damascena* = meaning from Syria; *bifera* = to split

*Rosa eglanteria* from French "eglantois" or sweet, thorny rose, a.k.a. *R. rubiginosa*

*Rosa eglanteria* = from the French, referring to this sweet, scented, thorny rose; a.k.a. *R. rubiginosa* = rust colored

*Rosa gallica officinalis*

*Rosa gallica officinalis* = French rose used officially

*Rosa rubiginosa*

*rubiginosa* = rust colored

*Rosa damascena trigintipetala*

from Damascus in Syria and *trigintipetala* = three petaled

**Rosehip Seed** or **Rosa mosqueta** = musky (***R. eglanteria***)

**Rosemary** (***Rosmarinus spp.***)

*Rosmarinus* = rose of the sea

**Rosemary** (***Rosmarinus officinalis*** )

*officinalis* = used officially in medicine

**Rosemary Verbenon** (***Rosmarinus officinalis CT verbenon***)

**Rosemary Borneol** (***Rosmarinus officinalis CT borneol***)

**Rosemary Cineol** (***Rosmarinus officinalis CT cineol***)

*Verbenon, borneol,* and *cineol* are the chemicals that make the chemotype

**Rose Geranium** - See **Geranium**

**Sage** (***Salvia officinalis***)

*Salvia* = well preserved, refers to medicinal properties; *officinalis* = a plant used medicinally

**Sage, Clary** - See **Clary Sage**

**Sage** (***S. lavandulaefolia*** )

*lavandulaefolia* = leaves like lavender

**St. John's Wort** (***Hypericum perforatum***)

*Hypericum* = the Greek word for upper, an icon, an image according to Linnaeus, it was hung above pictures to ward off evil spirits; *perforatum* = to perforate and refers to the foliage

**Sandalwood (*Santalum album*)**

*Santalum* = the Sanscrit name for the sandalwood tree; *album* = white

**Sassafras (*Sassafras albidum*)**

*Sassafras* = probably adapted by French settlers from an American Indian name; *albidum* = whitish, from the underside of the leaves

**Savory (*Satureia hortensis* and *S. montana*)**

*Satureia* = savory; *hortense* = that grows in the garden; *S. montana* = savory that grows wild in the mountains

**Spearmint (*Mentha viridas*)**

*Mentha viridas* = mint that is green

**Spikenard (*Nardostachys jatamansi*)**

*Nardostachys* = the Indian spikenard which yields a fragrant substance used for unguents, it grows like the ear of grain or a spike; *jatamansi* = an Indian name for this plant

**Spruce**

**Black Spruce (*Picea mariana*)**

*Picea* = spruce; *mariana* = named after Mary, Virgin mother of Jesus. It is commonly called Black Spruce because of a lichen that is dark to black in color and grows on this tree, giving this type of spruce forest a black color from a distance

**White Spruce (*Picea alba*)**

*Picea alba* = spruce that is white

***Tsuga heterophylla***

*Tsuga* = refers to larch, from a Japanese name; *heterophylla* = with variable leaves this tree is commonly called a spruce and is usually not used in aromatherapy.

**Star Anise (*Illicium verum*)**

*Illicium* = seductive, refers to the fragrance; *verum* = an adverb from verus, meaning true or genuine

**Styrax (*Liquidambar styraciflua*)**

*Liquidambar* = refers to the resin; *styraciflua* = an ancient name for a tree producing a fragrant gummy resin, called storax by Pliny and Vergilius Maro

**Tagetes (*Tagetes glandulifera*)**

*Tagetes* = a plant name said to be named after Tages, Etruscan

God, grandson of Jupiter, who sprang from the earth as a boy and taught the art of plowing to the Etruscans; *glandulifera* = refers to an acorn or a gland

**Tangerine (*Citrus reticulata, C. nobilis*)** See Mandarin

**Tarragon (*Artemisia dracunculus*)**

*Artemisia* = named after the Goddess Artemis; *dracunculus* = dragon

**Tea Tree (*Melaleuca alternifolia*)**

*Melaleuca* = refers to the black and white contrast of the peeling bark on trunks and stems; *alternifolia* = alternate leaves

**Terebinth (*Pinus spp.*)**

**Thuja (*Arbor vitae, Thuja plicata, T. occidentalis*)**

*Arbor vitae* = tree of life; *Thuja* = that is resinous and sweet-scented, named by Theophrastus, a fragrant tree with shoots that appear plaited or plate-like or in a flattened plane; T. *plicata* = with plaited leaves, from the west; *T. **occidentalis*** = fragrant tree

**Thyme**

**Thymus (*Thymus vulgaris*)**

*Thymus* = from the Greek word meaning the soul, mind, or will; *vulgaris* = common

**Lemon Thyme (*T. hiemalis*)**

*hiemalis* = belongs to winter

**Sweet Thyme (*T. vulgaris* CT linaloöl)**

**Red Thyme (*T. vulgaris* or *T. zygis*)**

*vulgaris* = common; *zygis* = from the Latin, zygo = meaning joined

**Oregano (*T. capitatus* )**

*capitatus* = has a head

**Oregano (*O. vulgare* )**

*Oregano* = Greek for mint; *vulgare* = a common plant that spreads itself out

**Marjoram (*Origanum majorana* )**

*Origanum majorana* = the larger form of the plant that spreads itself out

**Wild Marjoram (*Thymus mastichina*)**

*mastichina* = gummy

**Sweet Marjoram (*Majorana hortensis*)**

*Majorana hortensis* = a large plant or a major plant of the garden

**Thyme** (***Thymus vulgaris***)

*Thymus vulgaris* = common thyme

**Tuberose** (***Polyanthes tuberosa***)

*Polyanthes* = many or just separate-parted blossoms; *tuberosa* = tubelike

**Vanilla** (***Vanilla planifolia***)

*Vanilla* = a sheath or scissors case; *planifolia* = possibly from *planeta* or *planetum* or *plana* which means flat-leafed, wandering leaves

**Verbena** or **Lemon Verbena** (***Aloysia triphylla***)

*Verbena* = sacred boughs and plants used medicinally; *Aloysia* = after Maria Louise, Princess of Parma, died 1819; *triphylla* = leaves in whorls of three

**Vetiver, Vetivert, Khus-Khus** (***Andropogon zizanioides*** [***muricatus***])

*Andropogon* = a bearded male; *zizanioides* = darnel, the tares, the injurious weed of grain fields of Scriptural parable. Zizania is like Canadian wild rice

**Violet Flower** and **Leaf** (***Viola odorata***)

*Viola* = the violet; *odorata* = sweet smelling or fragrant

**Wintergreen** (***Gaultheria procumbens***)

*Gaultheria* = after Dr. Gaulthier (1708 - 1758), a Canadian botanist and physician; *procumbens* = falling forward or prostrate

**Yarrow** (***Achillea ligusticum*** and ***A. millefolium***)

*Achillea* = after the God Achilles, refers to the fact that this plant was used to heal his wounds; *ligusticum* = to bind with yarrow; *millefolium* = a thousand flowers

**Ylang-Ylang** or **Ilang-Ilang** (***Cananga odorata***)

*Cananga* = a Malayan name; odorata = the fragrant flower of flowers

"As you can see the 'whys' of these plant names are varied, many being implicitly named for a region or area where no doubt the plant was found. Other reasons why a plant might be given a certain name may be more arbitrary, based upon the preferences or idiosyncrasies of the taxonomist. Also, some plants are given Latinized names descriptive of their notable characteristics, e.g., three-leaved, etc."

— from Michael A. Flannery,
Library Director of the Lloyd Library,
1998.

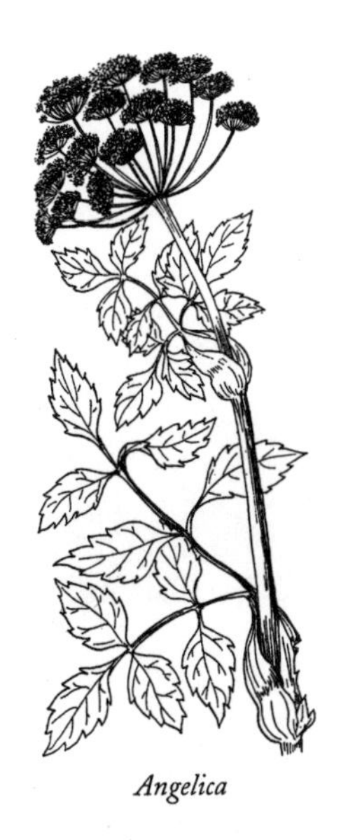
*Angelica*

# THREE

# Essential Oils Are More Than Stinky

Essential oils, which are harvested from various plant parts by distillation, are composed of many different components. The chemical ingredients give to each essential oil the scent of the essence. Some of these components have more odor than others, but the totality of the components are the eponymous scent or odor of the plant. By the nature of heat or steam (heat) and subjecting the plant to steam distillation, the odor of the resultant essential oil is not exactly the odor of the living plant. And distillation produces some ingredients in the essential oil that are not present in the living plant. As an example, one of these new components is the azulene produced by the destructiveness of the distillation of Chamomile.

Essential oils have scent, but they also have *color, viscosity,* and *taste.*

## Experience the Aromas

Just how do you describe an odor? This is not a simple task. We have plenty of words to describe the other senses of touch, hearing, and sight but scent is an experience bereft of words. These words you must make up yourself so that once an odor is smelled, absorbed by the nasal mucosa, and imprinted on your limbic system, it will be forever remembered.

***You Will Know Them by Their Scent***

Some of the words that are used traditionally in perfumery to describe odor and some of the plant scents that are representative are:

| | |
|---|---|
| Floral | can be Rose, Jasmine, Lilac, Orange flower |
| Fruity | can be Peach, Plum, Strawberry |
| Citrus | can be Orange, Lemon, Grapefruit |
| Conifer | can be Spruce needles, Fir needles, Pine |
| Minty | can be Spearmint, Peppermint |
| Green | can be Galbanum, Green Pepper, Green Peas |
| Vegetable | can be freshly sliced Potatoes, Cabbages, Carrots |
| Woody | can be Sandalwood, Cedarwood |
| Herbaceous | the scent of withered leaves, Thyme, Marjoram |
| Hay | the smell of the sun on warmed plants, Tonka beans |
| Smoky | smoldering leaves in the yard, castoreum |
| Leather | saddles, harness, and shoes |
| Powdery | traditional baby powder, soft and lightly fragrant |
| Fungal | dark and cool, undergrowth, Mushroom $CO_2$, or ripe mushrooms |
| Camphoraceous | smells like Camphor, Rosemary, Lavender Camphor |
| Earthy | warm earth, sun-baked soil, Patchouli, Oakmoss |
| Marine | seaweed, the sea, fresh ocean fish |
| Mossy | dried moss or lichens, chypre, Oakmoss, Treemoss |
| Oily/Fatty | Olive oil, any fatty oil |
| Aldehydic | synthetic, any of the new perfumes |
| Waxy | the smell of beeswax, paraffin |
| Honey | typical warm honey odor, Wallflowers |
| Civet | cat urine (very specific) |
| Musky | a clean, bright, sexy odor (an example is ambergris, an unknown (ambered) odor to most of us) |
| Balsamic | balsam of Tolu, Peru, or Benzoin |

| | |
|---|---|
| Caramel | burnt sugar, toffee, Tuberose absolute |
| Spicy | Cinnamon, Cloves, Nutmeg |
| Almondy | Bitter Almonds, Cherry kernels, Peach kernels |

Okay, now that you have the vocabulary, take each one of the oils that you possess and describe them using the above terms. Call this an Odor Profile. You should do one profile every morning upon awakening and then again in the evening using the same oil. You will note that your sense of odor changes throughout the day. Remember to do your odor profile in a clean, unscented space with only a bit of air flowing. For women, the perception of odor changes throughout her menstrual cycle, and women may want to repeat the Odor Profile on certain essential oils when they are menstruating. At this time, do an Odor Profile of Jasmine absolute, Rose, and Lavender, and note how different the scent is from your midcycle testing.

Repeat your sensory testing as often as possible until these 28 descriptive words are memorized.

There are other words, adjectives, to describe odors and blends and among these are *Anise-like, Animal, Burnt, Faecal* (Jasmine), *Forest, Metallic, Peppery, Tobacco.* There are words to describe the characteristics of odor such as *Balanced, Diffused, Dry, Flat, Fresh, Harmonious, Harsh, Hay, Light, Mellow, Musty, Rich, Rounded, Sharp, Smooth, Pointy, Sweet, Thin, Warm, Hairy, Nauseous*, and so on.

Now that you have a vocabulary to work with, go over each of the oils that you possess and write a sentence about each using your descriptive vocabulary and using these words that help you remember each and every scent.

### *Remember: Waft Don't Draft*

This means to wave the odor blotter or bottle under your nose rather than inhaling it in one long draught. The sweet, high notes are available from wafting (waving back and forth and taking short sniffs), while the heavy, composty notes come up when drafting (taking one long sniff straight from the bottle).

Remember that many essential oils have several different scents depending on chemotype. Lavender (*vera*) can be smooth, soft, and floral or heavy in camphor odor depending on whether it is a true high–grown Lavender or a "landscape" Lavender. Lavender oil from Provence–type plants can be camphoraceous and sharp, and Lavandin Grosso can be sweet, soft, and herbaceous. Make your own notes on odor for your own use.

## Experience the Color

Colors of essential oils range from clear like water (Peppermint, Eucalyptus) to various blues of the Blue oils, the pink of Calamintha, the brown shades of Patchouli or the greenish-brown of Spikenard, the golden tones of *Cedrus atlantica*, and the variety of pale yellows to orange, such as those occurring in Lemon or Orange Peel oil. And, don't forget the green oils of Geranium and Seaweed.

## Color Can Also be a Sensory Experience

Smell your essential oils and write down your sensory impression. With eyes closed, describe them as you would color. For example: Litsea scent might be described as lemon yellow, chrome yellow, pencil yellow, mustard yellow, egg-yoke yellow, or pale and creamy yellow. Yellow color is also considered energizing and refreshing and one that can stimulate appetite. Think of your essential oils in terms of pictures, colors, and emotions, and describe them.

Place one drop of essential oil on the blotter strip and inhale from the blotter, wafting the blotter under your nose. Do not inhale from the bottle, as your nasal mucosa will quickly become overstimulated and unable to sense anything. After inhaling quickly, write down your impressions. Make sensory descriptions as well as odor profiles. You will become more familiar with each oil that you use.

## Look at the Viscosity

Viscosity can range from not viscous and runny to the very viscous resinous oils.

## Take a Taste

And taste? Indescribable. But many restaurant reviewers do. Put a tiny dab on your fingertip and touch to your tongue. Try to describe the taste of the essential oil. Try a range of culinary oils from Cumin, Dill, and Black Pepper to strictly therapeutic oils such as Basil linaloöl or *Ravensara aromatica.*

Yes, essential oils are much more than just a scent or fragrance.

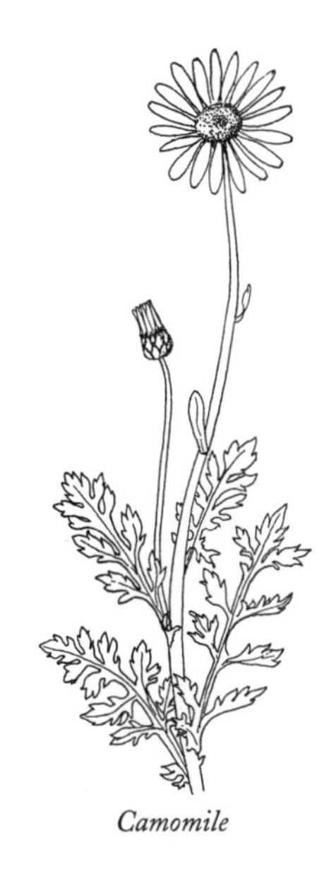
Camomile

# FOUR

# Botanical Classification of Essential Oil Plants

**Divsion:** ***Eumycetes (Thallophyta)***

Subclass: *Ascolichenes*

Family: *Usneaceae*

Genus: *Evernia*

**Divsion:** ***Embryophyta Siphonogama*** (seed plants)

**Subdivision:** ***Gymnospermae***

**Class:** ***Coniferae***

Family: *Podocarpaceae*

Genus: *Dacrydium*

Family: *Pinaceae*

Genera: *Picea*

*Tsuga*

*Pseudotsuga*

*Abies*

*Cedrus*

*Pinus*

Family: *Taxodiaceae*

Genera: *Sciadopitys*

*Cryptomeria*
*Sequoia*
Family: *Cupressaceae*
Genera: *Callitris*
*Thujopsis*
*Thuja*
*Cupressus*
*Chamaecyparis*
*Juniperus*
**Subdivision: *Angiospermae***
**Class: *Monocotyledones***
Family: *Poaceae*
Genera: *Elyonurus* (*Elionurus*, *Lygeum*)
*Vetiveria* (*Anatherum*, *Andropogon*)
*Cymbopogon* (*Andropogon*)
*Andropogon* (*Cymbopogon*, *Amphilophis*)
Family: *Cyperaceae*
Genus: *Cyperus*
Family: *Arecaceae*
Genus: *Cocos*
Family: *Araceae*
Genus: *Acorus*
Family: *Liliaceae*
Genera: *Allium*
*Lilium*
*Hyacinthus*
*Convallaria*
Family: *Amaryllidaceae*
Genera: *Narcissus*
*Polyanthes*
Family: *Iridaceae*
Genera: *Crocus*
*Iris*

Family: *Zingiberaceae*

Genera: *Hedychium*

*Kaempferia*

*Curcuma*

*Alpinia*

*Zingiber*

*Aframomum* (*Amomum*)

*Amomum*

*Elettaria*

**Class: *Dicotyledones***

Family: *Piperaceae*

Genus: *Piper*

Family: *Betulaceae*

Genus: *Betula*

Family: *Moraceae*

Genus: *Humulus*

*Cannabis*

Family: *Santalaceae*

Genus: *Osyris*

*Santalum*

*Fusanus*

Family: *Aristolochiaceae*

Genus: *Asarum*

Family: *Chenopodiaceae*

Genus: *Chenopodium*

Family: *Caryophyllaceae*

Genus: *Dianthus*

Family: *Ranunculaceae*

Genus: *Nigella*

Family: *Magnoliaceae*

Genus: *Magnolia*

*Michelia*

*Illicium*

Family: *Anonaceae*
  Genus: *Cananga* (*Canangium*)
Family: *Myristicaceae*
  Genus: *Myristica*
Family: *Lauraceae*
  Genera: *Cinnamomum*
    *Ocotea*
    *Sassafras*
    *Cryptocarya*
    *Laurus*
    *Umbellularia*
    *Aniba*
Family: *Brassicaceae*
  Genera: *Cochlearia* (*Armoracia*)
    *Brassica*
    *Raphanus*
Family: *Resedaceae*
  Genera: *Reseda*
Family: *Saxifragaceae*
  Genus: *Philadelphus*
Family: *Hamamelidaceae*
  Genera: *Hamamelis*
    *Liquidamber*
Family: *Rosaceae*
  Genera: *Spiracea*
    *Rosa*
    *Prunus*
Family: *Fabaceae*
  Genera: *Acacia*
    *Copaifera*
    *Myroxylon*
    *Lupinus*
    *Genista*

*Spartium*
*Wisteria*
*Hardwickia* (*Oxystigma*)
*Myrocarpus*
Family: *Geraniaceae*
Genera: *Geranium*
*Pelargonium*
Family: *Zygophyllaceae*
Genus: *Bulnesia*
Family: *Rutaceae*
Genera: *Xanthoxylum*
*Ruta*
*Pilocarpus*
*Cusparia*
*Boronia*
*Barosma*
*Amyris*
*Clausena*
*Citrus*
Family: *Burseraceae*
Genera: *Boswellia*
*Bursera*
*Commiphora*
*Canarium*
Family: *Euphorbiaceae*
Genera: *Croton*
Family: *Anacardiaceae*
Genera: *Pistacia*
*Schinus*
Family: *Tiliaceae*
Genus: *Tilia*
Family: *Malvaceae*
Genus: *Abelmoschus* (*Hibiscus*)

Family: *Dipterocarpaceae*
  Genera: *Dryobalanops*
    *Dipterocarpus*
Family: *Cistaceae*
  Genus: *Cistus*
Family: *Violaceae*
  Genus: *Viola*
Family: *Myrtaceae*
  Genera: *Myrtus*
    *Pimenta* (*Myrtus, Eugenia*)
    *Eugenia* (*Caryophillus*)
    *Leptospermum*
    *Melaleuca*
    *Eucalyptus*
Family: *Apiaceae*
  Genera: *Coriandrum*
    *Cuminum*
    *Apium*
    *Petroselinum*
    *Carum*
    *Pimpinella*
    *Foeniculum*
    *Anethum*
    *Oenanthe*
    *Levisticum*
    *Angelica*
    *Ferula*
    *Peucedanum*
    *Daucus*
    *Crithmum*
Family: *Ericaceae*
  Genus: *Gaultheria*
Family: *Primulaceae*

Genus: *Cyclamen*

Family: *Oleaceae*

Genera: *Syringa*

*Jasminum*

Family: *Verbenaceae*

Genus: *Lippia* (*Aloysia*)

Family: *Lamiaceae*

Genera: *Rosmarinus*

*Lavandula*

*Nepeta*

*Salvia*

*Monarda*

*Melissa*

*Hedeoma*

*Satureia*

*Hyssopus*

*Origanum*

*Majorana* (*Origanum*)

*Thymus*

*Mentha*

*Perilla*

*Pogostemon*

*Ocimum*

*Mosla* (*Orthodon*)

*Pycnanthemum*

*Coridothymus* (*Thymus*)

Family: *Myoporaceae*

Genus: *Eremophila*

Family: *Rubiaceae*

Genera: *Gardenia*

*Leptactina*

Family: *Caprifoliaceae*

Genus: *Lonicera*

Family: *Valerianaceae*
Genus: *Valeriana* (*Patrinia*)
Family: *Asteraceae*
Genera: *Solidago*
*Erigeron*
*Blumea*
*Helichrysum*
*Inula*
*Tagetes*
*Santolina*
*Chamæmelum* (Anthemis)
*Achillea*
*Matricaria*
*Artemisia*
*Arnica*
*Saussurea*
*Tanacetum*

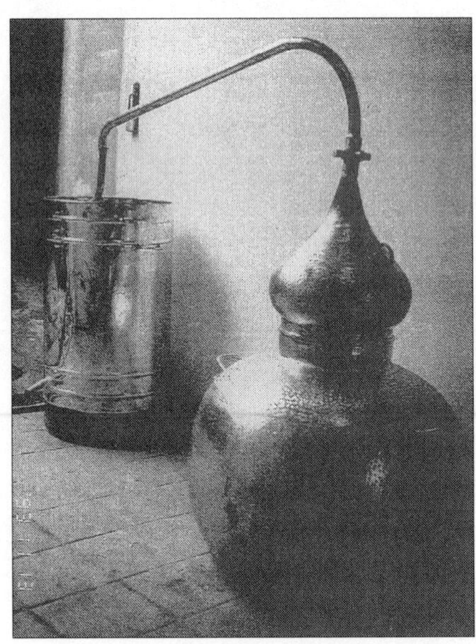

*Alembic still for Hydrosols*

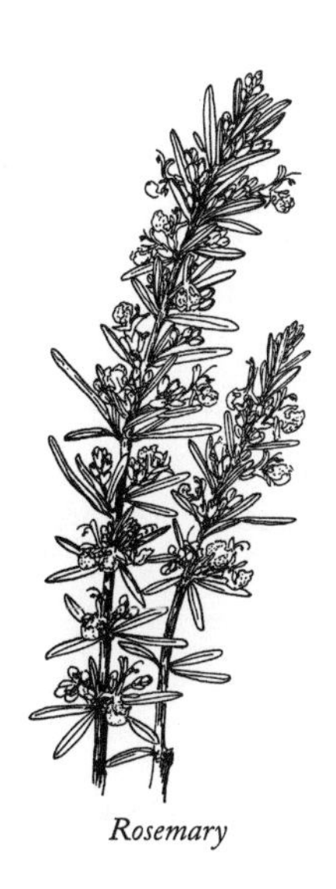
Rosemary

# FIVE

# Guide to Essential Oils

**Abbreviations Used Throughout**

| | | |
|---|---|---|
| S-D | Steam distilled | |
| AT | Aromatherapy | |
| EO | Essential Oil | |
| α/a/A | alpha | *variety of* |
| β/b/B | beta | *forms for* |
| γ/g/G | gamma | *components of* |
| δ/d/D | delta | *essential oils* |
| CT | chemotype | |
| HPA | hypothalamus/pituitary/ adrenal axis | |
| S-E | Solvent extracted | |

## Allspice *(Pimenta officinalis* or *P. dioica)*

*Family:* Myrtaceae

*Habitat & Growth:* Native to West Indies and South America. Cultivated in Central America. Evergreen tree 15 to 30 feet high.

*Scent:* Spicy and warm, like the spice.

*Components:* Berries, leaves occasionally S-D. Sesquiterpenes up to 7%; Phenols, mainly eugenol up to 90% among others.

*Properties, Indications, & Uses:* Anti-infectious, antibacterial, antiviral, antifungal, antiseptic, antiparasite, general stimulant, and aphrodisiac.

*Indicated for:* Dental infections, viral infections, bacteria in the colon, dysentery, sinusitis, bronchitis, colds, and flatulence.

*Uses:* Mainly used externally in massage. Also inhaled for respiratory system.

## Ambretta *(Hibiscus abelmoschus* or *moschatus)*

*Family:* Malvaceae

*Habitat & Growth:* Indigenous to India. Grown in other tropical countries. Evergreen shrub up to 5 feet.

*Scent:* Musky, spicy.

*Components:* Seeds S-D mainly in Europe. Sesquiterpenols, mainly Farnesol; Esters and Lactones, mainly Ambrettolide among other components.

*Properties, Indications, & Uses:* Hormone-like properties.

*Indicated for:* Certain hormonal insufficiencies.

*Uses:* Powerful adrenal stimulant. Can be used as an aphrodisiac or as an inhalant if one is trying to detoxify from steroid drugs.

## *Ammi visnaga* aka Khella

*Family:* Apiaceae

*Habitat & Growth:* Native to the Mediterranean and Western Asia. Annual herb, up to 2 feet, delicate leaves repeatedly divided, egg-shaped fruits.

*Scent:* Spicy, earthy, sharp, a mulchlike odor.

*Components:* Seeds S-D. Monoterpenes; Esters and Chromones, mainly 1% Khelline.

*Properties, Indications, & Uses:* Antispasmodic, coronary dilator, bronchodilator, and anticoagulant. Used as an inhalant to mask the function of the mast cells.

*Indicated for:* Insufficiency of heart muscle, atherosclerosis, asthma, colitis, liver disturbance, and allergic reactions.

*Uses:* Particularly useful in the treatment of respiratory problems, allergic asthma, and bronchial spasms.

*Contraindications:* Can cause photosensitization when used externally.

## *Amyris balsamifera* (West Indian Sandalwood aka Torchwood Tree)

*Family:* Rutaceae/No relation to Sandalwood

*Habitat & Growth:* Mainly Haiti, Venezuela, and other tropical areas. Small bushy tree.

*Scent:* Warm, woody, scent reminiscent of Sandalwood.

*Components:* Wood S-D. Up to 40% Sesquiterpenes; δ-Cadinene 16%, and the balance β-caryophyllene and others.

*Properties, Indications, & Uses:* Heart tonic and lymphatic and veinous decongestant.

*Indicated for:* Hemorrhoids and heart fatigue.

*Uses:* Mainly as a perfume fixative.

## Angelica *(Angelica archangelica)*

*Family:* Apiaceae

*Habitat & Growth:* Naturalized worldwide. Native to Europe and Siberia. A large biennial herb with large fernlike leaves. Flowers are borne on compound umbels.

*Scent:* Sharp, biting odor of green stems, just broken, with peppery overtones.

*Components:* Root and seed S-D. Root oil contains Lactones, Terpenes, mainly Phellandrene, Pinene and others. Seed oil is similar to the root oil but contains more terpenes such as β-Phellandrene and others.

*Properties, Indications, & Uses:* Nervous system sedative, carminative.

*Indicated for:* Spasms in the gut, anxiety, and nervous fatigue.

*Uses:* Oil of Angelica root and seed is contained in liqueurs such as Benedictine and Chartreuse as well as liquors like gin. It can be used to treat anorexia, asthma, and stomach ulcers.

## Anise seed *(Pimpinella anisum)*

*Family:* Apiaceae

*Habitat & Growth:* Naturalized worldwide. Native to Greece and

Egypt. An annual herb about 1 foot in height with fernlike delicate leaves and white flowers in umbels. Different botanically from Star Anise from *Illicium verum.*

*Scent:* Warm, sweet, licorice odor, like Italian Christmas cookies.

*Components:* Seeds S-D. Consists mainly of Anethole up to 90% and Methyl Chavicol among others.

*Properties, Indications, & Uses:* Estrogenlike properties, emmenagogue, aids childbirth, increases milk secretion, and antispasmodic for nerves and muscles. The French consider it psychoactive, carminative, tonic, and stimulant.

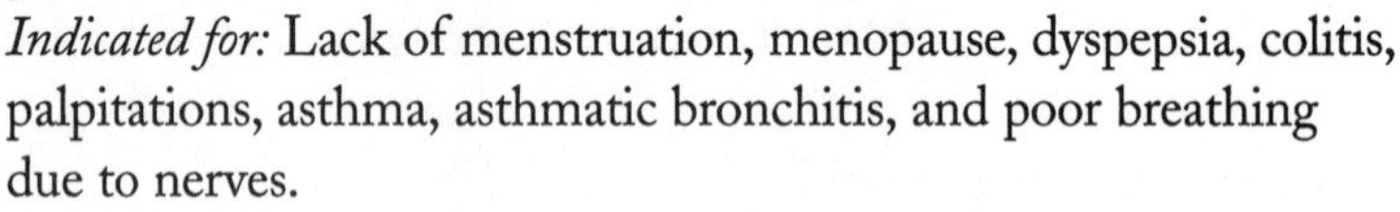

*Anise seed*

*Indicated for:* Lack of menstruation, menopause, dyspepsia, colitis, palpitations, asthma, asthmatic bronchitis, and poor breathing due to nerves.

*Uses:* Primarily in culinary preparations and mouthwash and to stimulate peristalsis.

### *Artemisia arborescens* aka **Great Mugwort or Blue Artemis**

*Family:* Asteraceae

*Habitat & Growth:* Grows well in all Mediterranean type climates. Cultivated mainly in Europe and Oregon. Perennial type herb up to 5 feet tall.

*Scent:* This is an indigo blue oil with a warm, smoky, and woody odor.

*Components:* Flowers S-D. Monoterpenes; high elevation of Azulene, an indigo blue oil called Blue Artemis. Sesquiterpene; Camphor up to 18%, among others.

*Properties, Indications, & Uses:* Mucolytic, anti-inflammatory, and antiallergenic, and has antihistamine qualities.

*Indicated for:* Mucus in the bronchial tubes, asthma, dermatosis, and serious skin infections or growths.

*Uses:* Can be used to treat eczema and psoriasis. Combine the essential oil in a 1% solution with *Aloe vera* gel to treat sunburn. Used neat to reduce raised moles.

*Contraindications:* Not to be used on babies, children, and pregnant women. Considered a neurotoxic and abortive.

***Artemisia douglasiana*** **aka White Sage or White Mugwort, the essential oil is called Blue Sage.**

*Family:* Asteraceae

*Habitat & Growth:* Grows wild in the northwestern United States.

*Scent:* This pale blue oil has a cooling, herbal, and eye-clearing odor with Sage and conifer notes.

*Components:* Tops S-D. Artemisia ketone and yomogi alcohol.

*Properties, Indications, & Uses:* Inhaled for mental states. Applied for muscular aches.

*Indicated for:* mental and physical conditions.

*Uses:* The herb is used in sweat lodges for cleansing the body and clearing the mind. The EO is used in blends for aching muscles and joints.

*Contraindications:* Do not use excessively.

**Balsam Peru (*Myroxylon balsamum* or *M. pereirae*)**

*Family:* Fabaceae

A different physiological form of Balsam Tolu.

*Habitat & Growth:* Native to South America. Tropical tree about 50 feet. The balsam is a pathological product from older trees.

*Scent:* Balsamic, healing, vanilla-type, warm, and smoky odor.

*Components:* Balsam is extracted by volatile solvents. Contains mainly Benzyl Benzoate; Benzyl Cinnamate (Esters up to 70%); an alcohol with a pleasant odor; Farnesol; Vanillin; and others.

*Properties, Indications, & Uses:* Anti-infectious, antibacterial, antiparasite, antiseptic, anticatarrh, expectorant, and cicatrix.

*Indicated for:* Bronchitis, chronic asthma, bad colds, virus, parasites, and skin disease.

*Uses:* Primarily used for skin care, the massage of muscles for circulation, and as an inhalant for respiratory and immune systems. Commercial use primarily in cough syrups and as a fragrance in soaps and lotions. Effective at relieving the itch of scabies, ringworm, pruritis, and eczema. It is also useful for relieving chapped hands and feet.

*Contraindications:* Prolonged skin use.

**Balsam Tolu (*Myroxylon balsamum*)** aka many synonyms

*Family:* Fabaceae

A different physiological form of Balsam Peru.

*Habitat & Growth:* Native to South America and different from Peru Balsam in that it branches 45 feet above ground.

*Scent:* Balsamic, healing, vanilla-type, warm, and smoky odor, like caramel.

*Components:* Balsam is S-D. A high Ester count, primarily of Benzyl Benzoate and Benzyl Cinnanate. Also Farnesol and others.

*Properties, Indications, & Uses:* Anticatarrh, expectorant, balsamic, urinary antiseptic, and anti-inflammatory.

*Indicated for:* Chronic catarrh, chronic purulent catarrh, chronic bronchitis, pneumonia, cystitis, prostatitis, and chronic inflammation of the urinary system.

*Uses:* Commercially used as a feeble expectorant in cough mixtures and as an inhalant for obstinate catarrh. Its vanilla-like fragrance contributes to its use in soap making and as a perfume fixative.

## Basil (*Ocimum basilicum*)

*Family:* Lamiaceae

The botanical classification of Basil is very complicated because of the many existing varieties and variety of forms. Basil is mainly divided into chemotypes of Camphor, Eugenol, Methyl Cinnamate, Rèunion, and Sweet Basil. Sweet Basil is often adulterated with other Basil. This increases the specific gravity and refractive index and lowers the laevo-rotation. The best way to identify these different oils is to purchase a little of each from various sources, smell them carefully, and learn to identify the different types simply by fragrance. The chemotypes (CT) may be identified by the increased amount of that particular chemical component in the oil. An example is the CT Methyl Chavicol type which contains up to 33% Methyl Chavicol, 40% Linaloöl, and 15% Methyl Cinnamate. These proportions will vary depending on habitat. A Citral type of Basil may produce up to 50% Citral, 15% Linaloöl, and very little Methyl Cinnamate. CT Camphor will produce up to 77% total components simply in Camphor.

*Basil*

*Habitat & Growth:* Indigenous to the Mediterranean area and grown in a variety of other countries, Basil is a small, compact annual herb. The entire plant is very fragrant with the typical eponymous scent of Basil.

*Scent:* Warm, spicy, and herbal with a hot, somewhat anise tasting "bite."

*Components:* Mainly Linaloöl with the CT presenting more or less amounts of the components after which it is named, among others.

*Properties, Indications, & Uses:* Generally used as an antispasmotic, anti-inflammatory, pain reliever, decongestant of the veins and pulmonary arteries, and antibacterial.

*Indicated for:* Insufficient digestive enzymes, pancreatic enzymes, urinary infections, congested prostate, rheumatoid arthritis, and viral infections. Pénoël and Franchomme mention six varieties of Basil with a variety of therapeutic uses. Some varieties of Basil are extremely caustic to the skin if applied neat.

*Uses:* A wonderful addition to many perfume blends, it works as a brain and memory stimulant and soothes stress, depression, and mental fatigue. The oil can be used in the bath. Another wonderful general use for Basil is with Rosemary verbenon as an external application on the hair and scalp to stimulate growth and condition hair.

**Exotic Basil (*Ocimum basilicum* var. *basilicum*)** Principle active components are 70–75% Chavicol and 12–14% Linaloöl. This Basil variation has action on the spinal bulb of the sympathetic nervous system. It is an anti-inflammatory when the inflammation occurs from an infectious origin, such as staphylococcus and pneumococcus.

*Indicated for:* Gas in the gut, problems of the prostate, urinary infections, and certain types of depression and fatigue.

**Lettuce Leaf** or **Large Leaf Basil (*O. b.* var. *"feuilles de laitue"*)** The principle components are alcohols, up to 65%, especially Linaloöl and Fenchol, aromatic Terpenes include Methyl-Cinnamate to 7%, Eugenol up to 12%. This type of Basil is used most often as a general stimulant for the digestive system and as a decongestant for the uterus or prostate.

*Indicated for:* Ulcers, prostatitis, uterine congestion, eczema, mental states such as depression and fatigue, and weakness or insufficiency of the cortico-adrenal gland.

**Green Basil (*O.b.* var. "*grand vert*")** The principle active components seem to be Methyl-Ether Phenols, especially Eugenol and Chavicol, with some 1,8-Cineol. This essential oil is considered strongly antispasmodic and anti-infectious.

*Indicated for:* Spasmodic colitis.

**Small Basil (*O.b.* var. *minimum*)** The active components are Eugenol and Chavicol. It is strongly antispasmodic and is used in much the same way as Green Basil.

**Other Basils**: Several other Basils are used in France in essential oil therapy. These include Camphor Basil, Eugenol Basil, and Thymol Basil.

**Camphor Basil** is mainly indicated for arterial hypertension and difficulties in circulation of the heart.

*Contraindicated:* For babies, children, and pregnant women.

**Eugenol Basil** seems to have hormonelike action on the prostate, is indicated for intestinal parasites, and is strongly caustic to the skin, so great care must be taken that it not be used neat on the skin.

**Thymol Basil** contains up to 47% Thymol and is contraindicated for external use as it is highly caustic to the skin; however, it is strongly anti-infectious and is considered a potent remedy for enterocolitis.

## Bay (*Laurus nobilis*)

*Family:* Lauraceae

*Habitat & Growth:* Mediterranean tree up to 60 feet in height.

*Scent:* Spicy, somewhat camphoraceous, herbaceous, and warm odor with a "bite."

*Components:* Leaves and branches S-D. Contains up to 50% Cineol and small amounts of Eugenol; Pinene and other components.

*Properites, Indications & Uses:* Expectorant and mucolytic.

*Indicated for:* Colds, virus infections, and mouth ulcers (aphtes).

*Uses:* Externally for massage in muscular aches and pains including arthritis. Can be inhaled in a blend for the respiratory system. Leaves are important culinary herb.

## Benzoin (*Styrax benzoin*)

*Family:* Styracaceae

*Habitat & Growth:* Native to Asia. Large tropical tree up to 60 feet high. Benzoin itself is the pathological product that forms when the bark is cut.

*Scent:* Sweet, warm-scented, brown balsamic resin with fragrance of spice and vanilla. Caramel, warm honey, a little waxy.

*Components:* Mainly Benzoic acid, 70% Benzoate, some Vanillin.

*Properties, Indications, & Uses:* Anticatarrh, expectorant, and pulmonary antiseptic.

*Indicated for:* Acne, eczema, psoriasis, and respiratory afflictions.

*Uses:* Inhalant for the respiratory system and preservative in food-stuffs. Used externally as a deodorant and antiseptic. When taken internally, it has an expectorant and diuretic effect.

## Bergamot (*Citris bergamia*)

*Family:* Rutaceae

Bergamot as a common name is also applied to an annual herb. These plants are in no way similar, and recently a company has supplied aromatherapy note cards with the fragrance of citrus Bergamot but a picture of the herb by the same name. Some believe Bergamot is a mutation of the sour Orange and not a hybrid. Bergamot Orange of the United States is cv. Bouquet.

*Habitat & Growth:* Native to Asia, naturalized in Italy, and grown commercially in several places. Delicate citrus tree approximately 12–15 feet in height. Small, round citrus fruits are often picked when green. The most delicate of all citrus plants, demanding special climate and soil.

*Scent:* Citrus spice with a high floral note.

*Components:* Oil of petitgrain Bergamot is occasionally produced. Oil from peel extracted by cold expression or vacuum distillation to produce a Terpene-free oil. The main component is Linalyl acetate, with free Linaloöl, varying from 20–30%, among others. Ester content changes depending on climate in that year.

*Properties, Indications, & Uses:* Calming and anti-inflammatory. Used by application for a variety of skin problems. Used by inhalation for anxiety and depression. Used as a gargle for a sore throat.

Application methods include lotion, compress, bath, salve, unguent, sitz bath, and massage.

*Indicated for:* Depression, stress, and insomnia.

*Uses:* Inhaled for depression, stress, and insomnia. Applied externally in massage. Treats a variety of skin conditions, including acne, cold sores, herpes, eczema, psoriasis, and skin infections. Very important in perfume industry. Unripe fruits are preserved in Greece as sweetmeats to be eaten by the spoonful when having coffee or as a dessert.

## Birch Bark (*Betula lenta*)

*Family:* Betulaceae

*Habitat & Growth:* Native to Canada and United States. Lovely tree with a pyramid shape about 75 feet in height. The bark is a peeling bark. Birch tar oil is produced from *Betula alba* and used for chronic skin disease.

*Scent:* Sweet, spicy, and minty odor, a wintergreen chewing gum odor.

*Components:* Bark macerated in water and then S-D produces an EO up to 98% Methyl Salicylate among other components.

*Properties, Indications, & Uses:* Anti-inflammatory, antipyretic, antiseptic, astringent, and tonic.

*Indicated for:* Massage for rheumatism. Inhaled for hypertension.

*Uses:* Flavor for gum and toothpaste. It is a counter-irritant, so good for muscular aches and strains. It can also be used as a diuretic for water retention and edema.

*Contraindications:* Skin irritant and marine pollutant.

## Black Pepper (*Piper nigrum*)

*Family:* Piperaceae

Not to be confused with Chilé Pepper or Cubebs. Black Pepper berries are one of the most important and oldest spices known, having been used and noted in Greek herbals to 500 BC. It was occasionally used as trade money. Toward the end of the 15th century, Vasco da Gama discovered the water passage to the Malagar Coast which was one of the principal spice-producing territories at that time. With the discovery of the sea passage, the modern spice trade came into being.

*Habitat & Growth:* Native to India. Cultivated extensively in various parts of the world. Perennial, woody vine that produces small berries that blacken when they mature.

*Scent:* Hot, sharp, bright, fruity, and spicy odor.

*Components:* Berries are crushed and S-D to produce a slightly greenish EO with a powerful pepper scent and with no taste. The flavor of Black Pepper that causes digestive disturbance does not occur in the EO. Contains Phellandrene and Pinene among others.

*Properties, Indications, & Uses:* Anticatarrh, expectorant, gland stimulant, and aphrodisiac.

*Indicated for:* Toothache, laryngitis, chronic bronchitis, rheumatism, and sexual debility.

*Uses:* Wonderful ingredient in culinary aromatherapy; used especially when the pungency of Black Pepper berries causes *digestive* distress.

**Blue Artemis**

(See *Artemisia arborescens*)

**Blue Chamomile**

See **Camomile.**

**Blue Cypress (*Callitris intratropica*)**

*Family:* Cupressaceae

The jewel of Australian essential oils.

*Habitat & Growth:* Native to Australia. A tree that is shrublike in shape. The bark is peeled, and what is left is S-D to produce a deep-blue viscous oil.

*Scent:* Deep, woody, and like Juniper berries and Cypress.

*Components:* Wood oil contains guaiol, guaienes, selinenes, guaiazulene, eudesmols, and furanones.

*Properties, Indications, & Uses:* Anti-inflammatory, antihistamine, and antiviral. An excellent fixative. Used in perfumery as a base note.

*Indicated for:* Arthritis and asthma.

*Uses:* Inhaled for allergic asthma, because guaiazulene is proven to limit histamine production, and anti-inflammatory for arthritis.

**Blue Sage**

(See *Artemisia douglasiana*)

## Blue Tansy (*Tanacetum annuum*)

*Family:* Asteraceae

This lovely blue EO is incorrectly identified by many other names. It is an annual tansy that grows in Morocco.

*Habitat & Growth:* Native to Morocco and Southwest Europe. An annual herb that is greenish and somewhat hairy. The flowers are hermaphrodite. Occurs in cultivated ground and waste places.

*Scent:* Richly scented of toast and herbs. Deep indigo blue colored oil.

*Components:* Azulene and limonene.

*Properties, Indications, & Uses:* Hormone-like action, anti-inflammatory, antiphlogistic, antihistamine, and analgesic.

*Indicated for:* Asthma and skin care.

*Uses:* Nerve sedative, couperose skin, neuritis, sciatica, possibly stimulates the thymus, and may supply theophylline for adults and infants.

*Contraindications:* Not to be used on certain women with endocrine imbalance.

## Borneol (*Dryobalanops aromatica*)

*Family:* Dipterocarpaceae

I have been looking for this substance for a number of years and have never seen the true natural substance, nor have I ever known anyone else to have seen or used it.

*Habitat & Growth:* Native to Sumatra and Borneo. Tall majestic tree.

*Scent:* Like camphor and mothballs.

*Components:* Crystalline Borneol which occurs in the crevices and fissures of old trees. 35% Terpenes, primarily Pinene and Camphene; 20% Sesquiterpenes; and 25% resin; and 10% alcohol primarily δ-Borneol among others. Borneol is now primarily a synthetic material.

*Properties, Indications, & Uses:* Were it possible to be found, the natural substance is used as a stimulant to the adrenal cortex.

*Indicated for:* Adrenal weakness, fainting, and externally on abscess, herpes, ringworm, and boils.

*Uses:* "Among the Malayan and Chinese population of the Far East, Borneo Camphor is highly esteemed for embalming and ceremonial purpose."[1]

---

[1]Ernest Guenther, *The Essential Oils,* Vol. V (Malabar, Fla: Kreiger Publishing, 1976) p. 261.

## Cabreuva (*Myocarpis frondosus*)

*Family:* Fabaceae

*Habitat & Growth:* South American legume. A tall tree, 30 to 50 feet in height.

*Scent:* Softly floral and fruity. A pale yellow oil.

*Components:* S-D of wood. Farnesol, Sesquiterpene, alcohols, other components, mainly Nerolidol, up to 80%, among others.

*Properties, Indications, & Uses:* Hormone-like with possible action on hypothalamus. Aphrodisiacal and possible corticosteriod action.

*Indicated for:* Sexual debilities and various types of arthritis.

*Uses:* Scenting soap.

## Cade (*Juniperis oxycedrus*)

*Family:* Cupressaceae

See Evergreen

*Habitat & Growth:* Native to France and common in Europe. The tar is produced mainly in Spain and Yugoslavia. A large evergreen shrub, up to 12 feet.

*Scent:* A black tar with an oily, leathery, black smoke odor.

*Components:* Produced by destructive distillation of this particular Juniper. Process is called empyreumatic or partly decomposed. Also called Juniper tar. Sesquiterpene called Cadinene; Hydrocarbons and Phenols, among them Creosol.

*Properties, Indications, & Uses:* Skin disease, eczema, and severe dandruff.

*Indicated for:* Bad skin and greasy hair.

*Use:* In therapeutic soaps for chronic eczema. Used in ointments and salves for a variety of skin problems, including psoriasis.

There is also a true EO from S-D of the bark.

## Cajeput (*Melaleuca leucadendron* and *M. cajuputi*)

*Family:* Myrtaceae

Part of the group of plants called Tea Trees. The Melaleucas have great value in skin care and for wound cleansing.

*Habitat & Growth:* Grows wild in Indonesia and cultivated in other tropical countries. Tall evergreen, up to 90 feet. Part of the Tea Tree group of EO, the bark of which peels off.

*Scent:* A peculiar, musty, feet-sealed-in-socks odor, but less pungent than other Melaleucas.

*Components:* S-D of fresh leaves and twigs. Cineol, Pinene and Sesquiterpenes including Cadinene among other components.

*Properties, Indications, & Uses:* Anti-infectious, antiseptic, and hormone-like.

*Indicated for:* Genital herpes, respiratory infections, hemorrhoids, and varicose veins.

*Contraindications:* Not to be used on pregnant women.

## Calamintha (*Calamintha officinalis*)

*Family:* Lamiaceae

*Habitat & Growth:* Native to Europe, naturalized throughout the Americas. A bushy perennial about 3 feet in height.

*Scent:* Sharp, aldehydic, fruity, and minty. A yellow to pink colored oil.

*Components:* S-D of the tops produces a pinkish colored oil. Citral, Citronellol, and others.

*Properties, Indications, & Uses:* Tonic for respiratory and nervous system, liver stimulant, anti-infectious, antifungal, hormonelike, and *reduces* thyroid output.

*Indicated for:* Slow digestion, colitis, hyperthyroidism, and problems in respiratory system.

*Uses:* Wildcat lure because of content of Metabilacetone.

*Contraindications:* Not to be used on children and pregnant women.

## Calamus (*Acorus calamus*)

*Family:* Araceae

*Habitat & Growth:* Swamps in North America. Naturalized in Europe. Aquatic plant.

*Scent:* Smells of root and swamp, fatty, slightly fruity, and heavily sweet. A deep yellow to reddish oil.

*Components:* Rhizome S-D for a very sweet eponymous scent; Pinene, Camphene, Cineol, Beta-asarone, etc.

*Properties, Indications, & Uses:* Anticonvulsant, antiseptic, antibacterial, expectorant, and stimulant.

*Uses:* Root used in potpourris and antismoking mixtures, though *oil* has no home use. Used often in perfumery.
*Contraindications:* Oral toxin. Highly toxic.

### Calendula (*Calendula officinalis*)

*Family:* Asteraceae
*Habitat & Growth:* Native to Europe. Naturalized throughout the world. Annual herb up to 2 feet in height.
*Scent:* A rich toasty, balsamic odor. A golden yellow infused oil.
*Components:* Flower heads are infused with oil or extracted by solvent extraction. Calendulin, waxes in absolute. The essential oil of Tagetes, sometimes called Calendula oil contains Tagetone among other components.
*Properties, Indications, & Uses:* Used universally for all sorts of skin conditions. The infused oil is especially valuable as a carrier oil in AT products. Nourishes dry skin for a relaxing or soothing massage.

### *Calophyllum inophyllum* (aka **Kamani Tree, True Kamani, Alexandrian Laurel**)

*Family:* Clusiaceae
In Madagascar this oil is called Foraha or Vintanina. There are many names the oil is called. Dilo oil from the nuts and the nuts are called Punnai Nuts in Hawaii. The nuts are also collected in Ceylon and have another name.
*Habitat & Growth:* Native to India, naturalized to Hawaii. Sacred to Polynesians (mentioned in many old Hawaiian chants). Grows to 60 feet. Seeds dispersed by bats and by sea movement. Seeds germinate well in muddy and saline soils. Full grown tree has a thick trunk covered with a black, cracked, and gnarled bark, growing to a height of 2 to 3 meters with big, twisted branches. Firm, shiny leaves, and produces flowers with a sweet aroma, reminiscent of Lime. Yellow, apple-flavored fruit covers a nut which has a thick shell covering a pale yellow kernel. Considered a sacred tree by the tropical populations, it was planted surrounding royal marshes. When the areas were converted to Christianity, tree population dropped by the thousands.
*Scent:* Wood, rooty vegetables, fatty, and earthy. A dark, viscous oil.
*Components:* The vegetable oil is cold-pressed from the fruit and

In 1934, *Calophyllum* was prepared with ethyl ether and injected to treat leprous neuritis. Since this time, the oil of the seeds was tested on various skin problems and disorders.

A gangrenous sore of the leg of a 57-year old woman which required amputation was treated with the oil, and healing took place after 7 months. The oil was used to treat a young teenage girl whose leg had been crushed 4 years before by a cart with iron wheels and on whom grafts had failed. New grafts were attempted and after a treatment for 10 days with *Calophyllum* oil the 12 grafts worked perfectly, the wounds closed and the girl was cured within 2 months after admission.

Burns treated with *Calophyllum* have showed good results. Burns cured include: burns to the face from phosphorus; burns to the head from a pot of boiling milk; burns to the hands from a batch of caustic soda; burns to the scalp from boiling water and burns to the popliteal (back of the knee) from inflammable oil. The principle use of the oil is for radiodermatitis and has been used by dressings to heal lesions from ray therapy.

Before surgical treatment, the oil has been applied to recent anal fissures with success. Post-surgical treatments brought about sedation of pain and resorption of tissue on treatment after breast surgery, crushing of the leg, and two thigh amputations in which the femurs were visible over a length of 4 cm.

The healings of varicose ulcerous wounds, leprous wounds, especially when the wound is infected or becomes eczematous are considerably slower and the wounds must first be treated with Hexomedine or Neomycin compresses.

*—from Prima Fleur informative flyer, 1998 (see source list)*

seed together. It contains Stigmasterol and about 7% wax. Balsam, calophyllolide and calophyllic acid contained in the oil are thought to be connected to its curative effects.

*Properties, Indications, & Uses:* Analgesic, anti-inflammatory, and antibiotic properties. Indicated for: used successfully on mucosa lesions as well as on the epidermis. Used to cure chapped feet and hands, chilblain and skin cracks, vaginitis, erosions and ulcerations of the cervical matrix, and breast cracks.

*Uses:* Medicinal uses for hair and scalp, eczema, psoriasis, and facial neuralgia. In its native habitat, plant and oil have been used medicinally to treat a variety of ailments, mostly skin related. Leaves are calmative in skin and ocular infections. A hot bath for 30 minutes has proven useful in the treatment of dermatosis, urticaria, and eczemas. Maceration of the young leaves in water is used as an eyewash to kill the pain of irritated eyes. Young shoots are used with other plants internally and externally for treatment of burns, as well as the treatment of hernias. Oil or a plaster of fresh, crushed seeds diluted in sterilized coconut oil contains cicatrization properties and is used for scabs, varicose ulcers, fistulas, leprous ulcers, and burns. The oil of *Calophyllum* easily saponifies and produces an abundant lather on contact with sea water. The oil is analgesic and is used for sciatica and rheumatism. The pulverized seeds have been used to cure ulcers and bad wounds.

*Calophyllum* is used as a treatment for various problems of the hair and scalp, and for eczema, psoriasis, and facial neuralgia. The essential oil of *Ravensara* and the vegetable oil of *Calophyllum* have been studied together by Dr. D. Pénoël and mentioned in Phytomedicine, 1981 as a treatment for shingles (zona) and has been shown to have pronounced amelioration of the problem. A good mixture would be 25% Calophyllum vegetable oil, 25% Walnut oil, 40% Jojoba unrefined oil, and 10% Ravensara essential oil. Mix these together, label your container, and apply to the scalp (or skin problem) night and morning. You could also use 50% Calophyllum, 40% olive oil, and 10% *Ravensara.* The bark also has medicinal uses as an infusion or in other herbal remedies.

## Camomile (*Matricaria recutita*)

*Family:* Asteraceae

There is much discussion in the botanical world regarding the nomenclature and correct name for the two varieties of Camomile called German, Hungarian or Blue Camomile *(Matricaria recutita)* and Roman or English Camomile *(Chamaemelum nobile).* The Lewis'[2] believe these two plants to be identical in two morphological forms: the annual and perennial.

[2]Lewis, Walter H. "Notes on Economic Plants." *Economic Botany,* 1992: 426-430.

**The Blue Oils© by Jeanne Rose**

| Latin Name | Other Names | A/P | EO Color | EO Aroma | Major Components | EO Uses |
|---|---|---|---|---|---|---|
| *Chamaemelum mixtum* | Yellow chamomile<br>Ormenis multicaulis<br>Ormenis mixta, mixtum<br>Anthemis mixta<br>Wild Chamomile<br>Moroccan Chamomile | A | golden yellow | spicy, fruity | alcohol | all problems of liver & stomach, including parasites, serious skin disease |
| *Chamaemelum nobile* | Tea chamomile<br>Sweet Chamomile<br>Roman Chamomile<br>English Chamomile<br>Anthemis nobilis<br>Nobel Chamomile | P | very pale blue to clear | sweet, herby, no tenacity | esters | asthma, oral uses. Best for all uses |
| *Matricaria recutita* | Blue Chamomile<br>Wild, Small Chamomile<br>Matricaria chamomilla<br>German chamomile<br>Hungarian Chamomile<br>Sweet false Chamomile | A | deep blue | fruit & toasted nuts | azulene, bisabolene, bisabolol | anti-inflammatory, all skin care |
| *Artemisia arborescens* | Blue Artemis<br>Greater Mugwort | P | deep blue | Worm-wood-like | thujone, azulene | anticatarrh, skin care |

**The Blue Oils© by Jeanne Rose, *cont'd.***

| Latin Name | Other Names | A/P | EO Color | EO Aroma | Major Components | EO Uses |
|---|---|---|---|---|---|---|
| *Artemisia douglasiana* *var. of A. vulgaris* | Blue Sage | P | deep teal blue | sage & conifer | Artemisia, Ketone, Yomogi, alcohol | anti-inflammatory, Muscular aches and pains |
| *Tanacetum annuum* | Blue Tansy Moroccan Blue Chamomile | A | deep blue | toasty odor & warm flavor | azulene, limonene | hormone-like, skin, asthma |
| *Tanacetum vulgare* | Common Tansy many chemotypes | P | yellow to very pale watery blue | Worm-wood-like | up to 60% thujone | *No use in aromather-apy* |
| *Callitris intratropica* | Blue Cypress | Tree | viscous azure blue | woody, like Cypress | guaiazulene, eudesmol, selinene | anti-inflammatory, skin, asthma |
| **Others** | | **See *World of Aromatherapy*, p. 200-210** | | | | |

*A=Annual P=Perennial

*Oxidation changes the chemical composition of the essential oil. If any of these oils are greenish-black when they should be deep blue, it indicates oxidation, age, and the existence of free radicals, and they *should not be used* for therapy; furthermore, if the clear to yellow oils appear deep yellow to deep brown, they too have oxidized and are too old to use therapeutically.

*All of these essential oils are produced by steam distillation, which also results in the production of azuline.

They have found no morphological differences, saying that one is just a double form of the other. Other scientists totally disagree and refute this. Camomile has been discussed at great length in every AT book, including *The Aromatherapy Book: Applications & Inhalations*, pages 77–80. An extensive essay is in *World of Aromatherapy*, pages 200–210.

*Habitat & Growth:* Naturalized all over the world, native to Europe. The annual form is a single flower that grows to 1 foot in height; the perennial is a mat-like double that stays close to the ground.

*Scent:* German is a dark blue oil with a floral, vegetable, fatty, herbaceous, earthy, spicy scent. The Roman is a pale blue to clear oil and smells floral, fruity, aldehydic and sweet.

*Components:* The flower produces the best quality essential oil early in the morning. *Matricaria recutita* is deep, dark blue in color, containing large quantities of Chamazulene, Farnesene, and Bisabolol among other components. *Chamaemelum nobile* is a pale blue oil that turns yellow, containing mainly Esters among other components. See chart p. 58.

*Properties, Indications, & Uses:* Mainly an anti-inflammatory whether used internally or externally. Hormone-like and antispasmodic.

*Indicated for:* All kinds of skin disease and menstrual problems. Franchomme divides the plants and uses *C. nobile* for asthma and intestinal parasites and uses *M. recutita* primarily for infectious skin disease, eczema, and stomach distress.

*Uses:* Tea used as digestive tonic and anti-inflammatory.

## Camphor (*Cinnamomum camphora*)

*Family:* Lauraceae

The tree that produces Camphor comes in several varieties. var. *Pharmosana*, var. *Glaucescens*, var. *Linaloölifera*, and var. *Nominale.*

Camphor production is very big in Asia, although much Camphor produced today is synthetic.

*Habitat & Growth:* Generally cultivated in Asia. This is a large, tall evergreen tree up to 90 feet, producing a crystalline substance from the wood of mature trees. The true Camphor tree is called Hon-sho although other morphologically distinct varieties exist, as already described.

*Scent:* Spicy, herbal, and mothball-like odor.

*Components:* S-D from wood. Leaves and stalks contain: Camphor, L-Linaloöl and other components. Roots are mainly Safrol, some Camphor, alcohols, and Esters among others. When the crystalline substance is S-D, it produces Camphor oil which contains 50% Camphor, some Piperitone, and Cineol. (There is a 100 page monograph on Camphor in Guenther's *Essential Oils, vol. IV.)*

*Properties, Indications, & Uses:* Tonic, general stimulant, and in larger doses a cardiac excitant.

*Uses:* As a painkiller for rheumatism and neuralgia. Inhaled for catarrh and bronchitis. *Glaucescens* has few contraindications and is anti-infectious, antiviral, antifungal, and a general stimulant. Used primarily externally in massage or inhaled for the respiratory system.

*Contraindications:* Not to be used on babies and pregnant women.

### *Cananga odorata*

*Family:* Anonaceae

Since this is closely related to true Ylang-Ylang and rarely available on the open market, we will discuss it in the section on Ylang-Ylang. The oil is made by S-D and used in perfumery.

*Habitat & Growth:* Native of Molucca. Occurs wild and may obtain the height of 160 feet.

*Scent:* Sweet and floral odor with a little bit of citrus.

### *Cannabis sativa*

*Family:* Moraceae

There is only one other oil in this family that is used which is Hops.

*Habitat & Growth:* Plant being grown for its fiber and intoxicating properties.

*Scent:* Grassy, herbaceous, and intoxicating.

*Components:* Monoterpenes up to 16% including Pinene and Myrcene. Sesquiterpenes including Caryophylline 35%, Humulene up to 12%, and other components.

*Properties, Indications, & Uses:* Anti-inflammatory and decongestant.

*Indicated for:* Inflammation of the respiratory tree and the digestive tube.

*Uses:* The leaf is smoked to ease the pain of cancer, the nausea of radiation treatment, and to encourage appetite in those who are asthenic.

### Caraway (*Carum carvi*)

*Family:* Apiaceae

*Habitat & Growth:* Native to Europe and Asia. Naturalized in many places. A biennial herb up to 3 feet in height with fragrant seeds.

*Scent:* Herbaceous, spicy, celerylike, and fruity odor. A pale yellow to reddish (when old) oil.

*Components:* Seeds S-D; principally up to 60% Carvone and some Terpenes namely δ-Limonene.

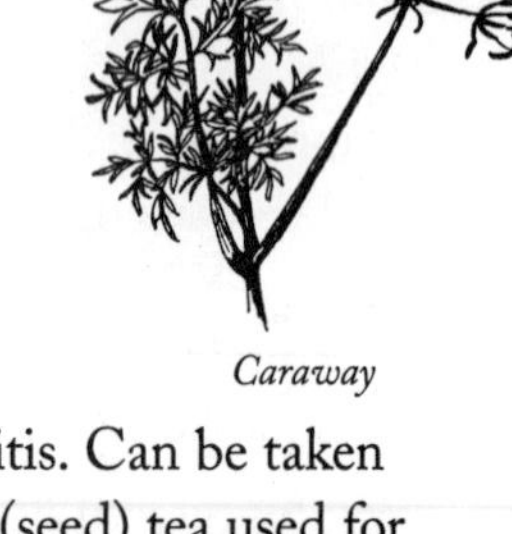

*Caraway*

*Properties, Indications, & Uses:* Mucolytic.

*Indicated for:* Respiratory system and liver.

*Uses:* Inhalant for chronic catarrh and bronchitis. Can be taken internally for insufficient liver and bile. Herb (seed) tea used for dyspepsia and stomachache. As a facial steam it can stimulate the complexion. It can be used on dogs to cure mange and scabies.

### Cardamom (*Elettaria cardamomum*)

*Family:* Zingiberaceae

Called True Cardamom

*Habitat & Growth:* Native to Asia, oil produced mainly in India. A perennial weed-like herb that grows up to 12 feet.

*Scent:* Distinctively spicy, fruity, warm, and balsamic odor. A golden yellow oil.

*Components:* Seed is distilled. Terpinyl acetate and Cineol, and terpenes.

*Properties, Indications, & Uses:* Tonic, stimulant, good for the stomach, eases gas pains, neuro-muscular, antispasmodic, expectorant, anti-infectious, antibacterial, antiparasite, and warming.

*Indicated for:* Digestive system, gut spasms, and inhaled for bronchial system.

*Uses:* Aphrodisiac mixtures. Spirit is used to flavor medicines.

## Carrot (*Daucus carota*)

*Family:* Apiaceae

*Habitat & Growth:* Native to Europe and Asia. Naturalized all over the world. Essential oil produced mostly in France. Annual or biannual herb with a tough but sometimes edible root. The top is called Queen Anne's Lace because of the lacy flowers. Grows up to 4 feet.

Scent: Herbaceous, mild, and spicy odor. A pale yellow oil.

*Components:* Seed EO obtained by S-D (occasionally used as part of an abortive procedure.) Pinene and Carotol, Limonene and Daucol among other components.

*Properties, Indications, & Uses:* Tonic, stimulant, liver regenerator, and control of cholesterol.

*Indicated for:* Insufficient liver, externally for skin problems, and to regulate the thyroid.

*Uses:* Oil used in flavoring liquors and in perfume compositions.

## Cedar

Cedar is a common name used for a variety of plants from family Pinaceae and family Cupressaceae. Family Pinaceae includes Atlas Cedarwood, Deodar Cedarwood, Lebanon Cedarwood, and family Cupressaceae includes Port Orford Cedar, Hinoki Cedar, Virginia Cedar, Texas Cedar, and others from the Juniper clan of this group of trees. All of the S-D Cedar oils are in general used externally, are well diluted for skin conditions, dandruff, fungal infections, and hair loss, and are inhaled in blends for the respiratory system.

## *Cedrus atlantica* Atlas Cedar See Evergreen

*Family:* Pinaceae

*Habitat & Growth:* Tall tree to 40 m. Natural habitat Atlas mountains of Morocco and Algeria.

*Scent:* A deep golden yellow oil. Woody and fruity with honey overtones.

*Components:* Yields 3-5% EO, cadinene, atlantone, and cedrol. Up to 80% Sesquiterpenes and Sesquiterpenols.

*Properties, Indications, & Uses:* Properties are arterial regenerative, a lymphatic tonic, aids in the removal of body fat. Indicated for arteriosclerosis, the retention of fluid in the tissue (edema), and externally for cellulite.

*Uses:* Inhale for respiratory problems, added to products for skin care and hair care.

*Contraindications:* See below.

A fragrant called "Cedarwood" actually from a Juniper (*Juniperus virginina*) is a wood used to line chests to repel vermin in the storage of valuables, especially furs and shoes. Cedar oil from *Cedrus spp.* can be used in the same manner. Care should be taken that garments do not directly touch wood treated with either of these oils called Cedar. *Contraindications:* Be aware of which Cedar you are using. Make sure you are using *Cedrus*, not *Juniperus* or *Thuja*. —*Jeanne Rose, 1994*

## *Cedrus deodora* Himalayan Cedarwood

*Family:* Pinaceae

See Evergreen, Chapter 6.

*Components:* Contains a quantity of Sesquiterpenes.

*Properties, Indications, & Uses:* Regenerates the arterial system. A lymphatic tonic, it is indicated for cellulite and water retention.

*Contraindications: Cedrus atlantica* and *deodora* are not to be used on children and pregnant women. Considered neurotoxic and abortive; however, I do not believe this.

## Celery (*Apium graveolens*)

*Family:* Apiaceae

*Habitat & Growth:* Native to Europe. Extensively cultivated. EO mainly produced in India. A biennial herb up to several feet in height.

*Scent:* The seed oil is pale yellow. Spicy, musky, and slightly vegetative odor.

*Components:* Seed is S-D or used in cooking. Herb used in food preparation. Root cultivated as well. Up to 60% Limonene with Selenine and Sesquiterpene alcohols among other components.

*Properties, Indications, & Uses:* Tonic, sedative, lymphatic drainage, and decongestant.

*Indicated for:* Asthenia, anxiety, and hemorrhoids.

*Uses:* Inhaled for respiratory system.

*Contraindications:* Some photosensitivity occurs when used externally.

## Champa, Champac (*Michelia champaca*)

*Family:* Magnoliaceae

An East Indian tree. The yellow flowers infused in oil yield a perfumed oil. The flowers are also worn in the hair. There is very little essential oil known. Essentially Yours, an essential oil company in England, has found a Champa that they feel sure has been distilled from the flower. Not much is known about the components. The incense called Champa is not from the flower and is probably totally synthetic.

*Scent:* Very sweet , rich, floral, and fruity odor with aldehyde, wax, and honey notes.

## Chilé (Red Pepper) (*Capsicum annuum*)

*Family:* Solanaceae

*Habitat & Growth:* Indigenous to the Americas. Medium-sized plant producing fruits of various size, color, and taste from sweet to *extremely* hot.

*Scent:* Hot, vegetative, and musty smell; it gives no indication of the burning sensation you would feel if you tasted it. A deep red oleo-resin.

*Components:* Oleo-resin of fruit prepared and then S-D. Contains mainly Capsaicin.

*Properties, Indications, & Uses:* This is a very concentrated oil. Used

as an animal repellant, it can be painted on the sidewalk to keep dogs from defecating on your property or painted on the fence to keep cats and deer out of your yard. Highly diluted in massage oil, it is great for improving circulation.
*Uses:* The pepper is excellent additive to the diet whenever there is respiratory distress or infection.

## Cilantro

See Coriander.
Prepared from the tops of the Coriander plant.

## *Cinnamomum spp.*

The French use a variety of Cinnamon in their therapy. They are all considered antispasmodic and anti-infectious. EO is used in respiratory blends, and the tea is used for colitis and spasm in the gut.

## Cinnamon (*Cinnamomum zeylanicum*)

*Family:* Lauraceae
*Habitat & Growth:* Native to Southeast Asia. Cultivated in other tropical countries. Tropical evergreen tree up to 45 feet high with small fragrant flowers and spicy, fragrant leaves.
*Scent:* Spicy, woody, with a bit of holiday and fruit scent, carries a sweet and biting note. A rich yellow oil.
*Components:* S-D from leaves and twigs and dried inner bark. Mainly Eugenol in the leaves and Cinnamaldehyde and Eugenol in the bark. Various types of Cinnamon produce various amounts of the components.
*Properties, Indications, & Uses:* Antispasmodic, anti-infectious, antibacterial, antiviral, and antifungal particularly against Candida and Aspergillis.
*Indicated for:* Tooth care, blends for vaginitis, impotence in men, respiratory blends for the lungs, and as a tea for sleepiness or depression.
*Uses:* Bark and leaf oils are in great use commercially in foods, mouth preparations, soaps, and toiletries.
*Contraindications:* This can be a very toxic EO and much care must be taken when using. **Skin irritant. Will cause erythema.**

**Cistus**

See Labdanum.

**Citronella (*Cymbopogon nardus*) [*C. Citratus* = Lemongrass]**

*Family:* Poaceae

Same genus as Lemongrass, Ginger grass, and Palmarosa grass.

*Habitat & Growth:* Native to Sri Lanka. Extensively cultivated in other tropical countries. A tall, perennial, aromatic grass.

*Scent:* Grassy, fruity, slightly herbaceous and bit of citrus odor. A yellow oil.

*Components:* S-D from above-ground parts. Among the components are Citronellal and Geraniol.

*Properties, Indications, & Uses:* Antispasmodic and anti-inflammatory.

*Indicated for:* Pelvic pain, rheumatism, and arthritis.

*Uses:* Good in blends for soaps and perfumes and for scenting rooms and repelling bugs. The oil can be used to clean and deodorize cooking surfaces. For example, use 5 drops of the EO and an ounce of vinegar as a wash for counters and stovetops.

**Citrus**

*Family:* Rutaceae

*Habitat & Growth:* A large group of EO producing plants. All parts of the tree produce EO. For example, Orange and Lemon trees produce Petitgrain oils from their leaves, called either Lemon Petitgrain or Orange Petitgrain. Orange flowers produce a hypnotic EO called Neroli. The fruit of Citrus produces delicious juices from the meat and EO that is expressed from the peel. The seed and pulp of Grapefruit and other Citrus fruits are also extracted to produce a Citrus seed extract that is used to preserve fine cosmetics.

*Scent:* Can only be described as citrus, smells like what it is, middle of forehead, clean and fresh.

*Components:* Citrus is a large group of essential oils, containing a variety of components, most particularly Geraniol, Linaloöl, and Limonene. For many more uses, look in your various aromatherapy books including my book, *The Aromatherapy Book: Applications & Inhalations*; Julia Lawless' *The Illustrated Encyclopedia of*

*Essential Oils*; Ernest Guenther's *The Essential Oils, vol. IV*; and Franchomme and Pénoël's *L'aromatherapie exactement.*
*Contraindications:* External use of many citrus oils can cause photosensitivity.

*Properties, Indications, & Uses* of many of the Citrus oils

***Citrus aurantifolia*** or Lime Peel oil: Soothing anti-inflammatory. Used for anxiety and stress.

***Citrus aurantifolia*** *ssp. aurantium,* called Orange Bigarade and Bitter Orange Peel oil: Calming and sedative. Used for anxiety and vertigo. The leaf oil is antispasmodic, anti-infectious, and used for nervous rheumatism, respiratory infections, and infected acne. The flower oil, Neroli, is primarily used for skin care, but has anti-infectious, neurotonic properties indicated for hemorrhoids, bronchitis, fatigue, and nervous depression. Neroli is one of the most important oils used in a diffuser for sweet, long sleep. The peel oil is a fragrant sweet addition to essential oil blends.

***Citrus bergamia*** or Bergamot peel oil: Anti-infectious, antibacterial, antiseptic, and tonic stimulant that is also calming and soothing. *Indicated for:* Poor appetite, insomnia, and agitation. Bergamot oil is one of our most important EOs to be used in blends. The small, sour fruit is also preserved in sugar and used as a sweetmeat with coffee. Petitgrain of Bergamot, from the leaves, is a calming anti-inflammatory indicated for stress, depression, and insomnia.

***Citrus hystrix,*** EO from Combava: Almost Clovelike scent. Anti-infectious, antiseptic, liver decongestant, neurotonic with hormonelike properties, and very calming.
*Indicated for:* Liver congestion and insufficiencies of the ovaries and testicles. Combava leaf oil is an anti-inflammatory and is a sedative indicated for anxiety, stress, agitation, and insomnia.

***Citrus latifolia,*** EO from Persian Lime peel: Sedative. Used for insomnia and anxiety.

***Citrus limetta,*** EO from Sweet Lime peel: Antispasmodic. Taken for spasms in the gut.

***Citrus limon,*** EO from Citron peel: Anti-infectious, antiseptic, antiviral, with action on the circulation and permeability of the capillaries. Calming for the nervous system, stomach, and most internal organs.

*Indicated for:* Respiratory infections, insufficient liver function, insomnia, nightmares, and disinfectant for air in the sick room for contagious ailments.

***Citrus medica var. vulgaris*** or Cedrat peel oil: Soothes stomach.

***Citrus paradisi*** or Grapefruit peel oil: Antiseptic for the air and disinfectant for any area where it is diffused. Also very important in skin care.

***Citrus reticulata var. mandarin*** or Mandarin peel oil: Moderates CNS symptoms. Relaxing and soothing.

*Indicated for:* Insomnia, pain, and gas in the gut. Somewhat helpful for dyspnea. Petitgrain or leaf oil is calming and is used for anxiety and stress.

***C. reticulata var. Tangerine:*** Same as Mandarin, but is grown in U.S.

***Citrus sinensis*** or Sweet Orange peel oil: Mainly antiseptic, calming, and sedative. Used to disinfect local areas. Inhaled for anxiety and nervousness. Wonderful in blends for a fresh, sweet scent.

***Citrus*** x spp. var. Clementine (Algerian mandarin): A cross between the sour orange and the mandarin. Most sold in the United States are imports from Spain. The Clementine is the parent of other hybrid mandarins, including the Fairchild and Robinson. A very rich, sweet Citrus scent, bright and sharp with a floral tone.

> "Clementines, also known as Algerian mandarins, are commonly believed to have been an accidental hybrid that was planted by the Reverend Clément Rodier around the turn of the century in the garden of the Catholic orphanage he ran in Algeria. Clementines are a cross between the sour orange and the mandarin. Most of the Clementines sold in the United States are seedless imports from Spain and are available from November to March. The Clementine hybrid is also the parent of other mandarin hybrids, including the Fairchild and the Robinson." —*Country Living, January 1996*

## Clary Sage (*Salvia sclarea*)

*Family:* Lamiaceae

*Habitat & Growth:* Native to Europe. Cultivated worldwide. Can be a very tall biennial or perennial herb up to 6 feet in height with large, hairy green leaves.

*Scent:* Woody green herbaceous and pleasant conifer odor that is mildly intoxicating.

*Components:* S-D from tops of plants, a concrète and absolute are obtained for the industry, produces by weight up to 0.14% EO. Up to 70% Ester, Linalyl acetate, Linaloöl, and others.

*Properties, Indications, & Uses:* Has estrogen-like properties useful in menopause, for hot flashes and as an aphrodisiac. Considered antispasmodic, reduces epileptic attacks, relaxing, and neurotonic.

*Indicated for:* Lack of menstrual cycle or scanty menstrual cycle, hemorrhoids, and nervous fatigue. Inhaled for hot flashes.

*Uses:* It can be gargled for a sore throat. The scent can help lift depression and soothe PMS (premenstrual syndrome) and emotional distress. It is mildly intoxicating and can create a sense of euphoria.

## Clementine

See Citrus.

## Clove (*Syzygium aromaticum*)

*Family:* Myrtaceae

*Habitat & Growth:* Cultivated worldwide. Evergreen tree up to 40 feet in height. Cloves used in commerce generally exported from Zanzibar. Originated in the Molucca Islands, but these Clove Trees were uprooted.

*Scent:* Warm, very spicy, and woody odor with a subnote of leather.

*Components:* S-D from the hand picked, unopened dry flower buds. 60–90% Eugenol among others.

*Properties, Indications, & Uses:* Anti-infectious, antifungal, and general stimulant.

*Indicated for:* Tooth problems.

*Uses:* Therapeutically to regulate thyroid and for some types of cancer. Uses are mainly in the commercial industry in dental preparations, candy, and gum.

*Other uses:* Clove fragments are added to Indonesian Kretek cigarettes.

*Contraindications:* Can cause serious skin and mucous membrane irritations. Julia Lawless states that "only the bud oil, and not the leaf or stem oil, should be used."

## Combava

See Citrus.

## Copaiba (*Copaifera spp.*)

*Family:* Fabaceae

The balsam Copaiba is the oleo-resin obtained from the trunk of various of these ssp. Mainly used as Copal resin in Mexico in incense.

*Habitat & Growth:* Native to the Amazon. Tall tree with a large trunk. Copaiba balsam also comes from other trees in Africa and other tropical countries.

*Scent:* Spicy, herbaceous, and warm tone with lots of high notes and a nutty side. Clear liquid that has a very mild, nonmemoristic scent and pale golden $CO_2$.

*Components:* Balsam of this rainforest plant is harvested by natives using a bamboo tube which is driven into a hole in the trunk. The balsam flows easily and is a clear liquid. This balsam is often adulterated with kerosene, turpentine and mineral oil. True Copaiba balsam contains a and b Caryophylline and other Sesquiterpenes.

*Properties, Indications, & Uses:* The French consider this a strong anti-inflammatory.

*Indicated for:* Urinary and pulmonary infections.

*Uses:* Extensive use in external and internal medicinal preparations. Considered a good fixative in soap scenting.

## Coriander (*Coriandrum sativum*)

*Family:* Apiaceae

The EO called Coriander oil is from the seed. The EO called Cilantro or Chinese Parsley is from the leaf of the Coriander.

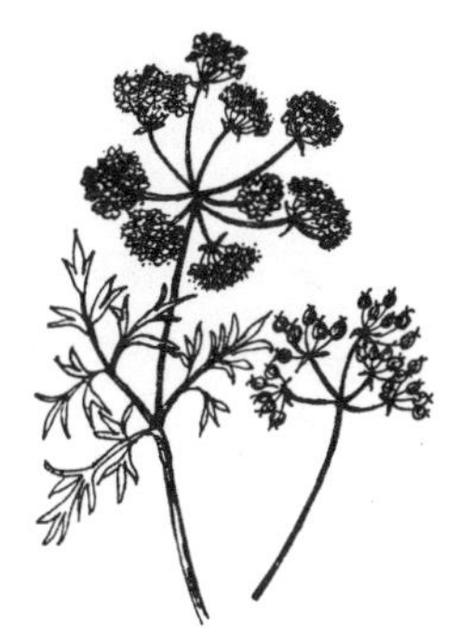

*Coriander*

*Habitat & Growth:* Native to Europe. An annual herb, strongly aromatic, and about three feet high.

*Scent:* Green, sharp, and smells like the herb Cilantro. Tastes soapy.

*Components:* S-D seed or leaf. Mainly up to 75% Linaloöl, among others.

*Properties, Indications, & Uses:* Anti-inflammatory and sedative.
*Indicated for:* Stress, anxiety, and insomnia.
*Uses:* Tea for stomachache or gastritis. Very important component in many EO blends because of its sharp, spicy note which is a welcome addition. Used as a massage oil to ease arthritis pain and migraine headaches. Can also be applied to clear blackheads and for oily skin.

## Costus (*Saussurea lappa*)

*Family:* Asteraceae

A tall, sturdy, herbaceous perennial up to eight feet high, large radical leaves, robust stem, and bearing a cluster of bluish-black flower heads.

*Habitat & Growth:* Indigenous to northwest regions of Himalayan Mountains. Locally called "Kuth." Thrives in shady, moist places beneath birch and dwarf willow at altitudes ranging from 9,000–11,000 ft.

*Scent:* Light-yellow to brown in color; peculiar animal-like lasting odor like violet, orris, and vetiver.

*Components:* Root is S-D. Yields viscous oil. Aplotaxene 20%, costus acid 14%, costol 7%, and a lactone, and others.

*Properties, Indications, & Uses:* Aphrodisiac, insect repellent, incense, and to perfume and preserve wool. Since ancient times used as aromatic stimulant against all disease.
*Indicated for:* Chronic coughs, cramps and gastric spasms.
*Uses:* In perfume in very small amounts.
*Contraindications:* Powerful skin sensitizer.

## Croton (*Croton eluteria*)

*Family:* Euphorbiaceae

Common name is Cascarilla, which is generally known as a bark with a fragrance much like Cinnamon bark.

*Habitat & Growth:* Indigenous to the Bahamas. Small tree or shrub. The bark is used with its aromatic odor and bitter, spicy taste.

*Scent:* Spicy, fruity, woody with a bite.

*Components:* On S-D the bark can produce up to 3% volatile oil. Containing a number of Sesquiterpenes and Monoterpenes.

*Properties, Indications, & Uses:* Eases pain along the nerves.

*Indicated for:* Headache.
*Uses:* Bark is sometimes used to flavor tobacco. The bark tea is sometimes used for stomachache.
*Contraindications:* Can be toxic when used orally, sometimes a skin irritant.

## Cubeb (*Piper cubeba*)

*Family:* Piperaceae
*Habitat & Growth:* Native to Indonesia. Evergreen vine up to 20 feet. Related to Black pepper. Not to be confused with *Litsea cubeba,* which is a shrub and not a vine.
*Scent:* Hot and spicy with a citrus note and a vegetable afternote.
*Components:* S-D from the unripe berries. Mainly Sesquiterpenes, among others.
*Properties, Indications, & Uses:* Anti-inflammatory
*Indicated for:* Urinary tract infections, cystitis, vaginitis, and externally for rheumatism.
*Uses:* Presently EO is not generally available.
*Historical use:* In the urinary system in the late stages of gonorrhea, as well as an inhalant to stimulate mucous membranes in the treatment of severe bronchitis.

## Cumin (*Cuminum cyminum*)

*Family:* Apiaceae
*Habitat & Growth:* Native of Turkey or Egypt. Grown heavily in the Mediterranean countries. Seed has been known since at least 2000 B.C. Slender, pretty, annual herb. Up to 1 foot in height.
*Scent:* Hits you in the stomach and makes your mouth water. Warm, spicy, nutty, and fatty.
*Components:* Plant contains up to 2.5% EO, S-D. Mainly 60% Aldehydes including Cuminaldehyde 35–65% and up to 52% Monoterpenes.
*Properties, Indications, & Uses:* Calming, stupefying, strong antispasmodic, and stimulating digestive.
*Indicated for:* Dyspepsia, gas and spasms in the gut, insomnia, hyperthyroid function, and orchitis.
*Uses:* Ritually used to protect the home and for internal protection. Recommended as a massage oil for poor circulation and lymphatic congestion.

## Cyclamen (*Cyclamen europaeum*)

*Family:* Primulaceae

Grows wild in Europe. Small pretty plant. Flowers are very sweet smelling and have been experimentally extracted as a pommade. An absolute was obtained. Contains Nerol and Farnesol. Not commercially produced.

## Cypress (*Cypressus spp.*)

*Family:* Cupressaceae

See Evergreen, Chapter 6

A variety of oils are produced that are called Cypress: oil from *Cupressus sempervirens,* Portuguese Cypress from *C. lusitanica,* Guatemala Cypress oil, Monterey Cypress from *C. macrocarpa,* Hinoki oil from *Chamaecyparis obtusa* containing 40% Terpenes and used extensively in Japan especially for the scenting of soap and in insecticides, Port Orford Cedar, and *Chamaecyparis lawsoniana* containing up to 46% d & a-Pinene.

## Cypress (*Cupressus sempervirens*)

*Habitat & Growth:* A tall evergreen tree native to the Mediterranean.

*Scent:* Clear, fresh, light, woody, oily, airy, and clean scent.

*Components:* 45% Monoterpenes and Sesquiterpenes such as 7% Cedrol.

*Properties, Indications, & Uses:* Anti-infectious, spasmolytic, and veinous decongestant.

*Indicated for:* Colitis or infections of the gut, decongest the prostate, and to stimulate the pancreas.

*Uses:* Another species of Cypress *(C. arizonica*)* is sometimes used in blends for massage to stimulate circulation and has particular use in reducing signs of cellulite. Julia Lawless uses Cypress oils in skin care for oily skin, in massage for rheumatism, poor circulation, as an inhalant for asthma and bronchitis, and for menstrual and menopausal problems. This oil is mostly used externally in massage, but can be taken internally with supervision. It is an astringent and can be used for oily hair and skin, as well as for sweaty palms. The fragrance is comforting and aids in

**Contraindications:* Pénoël considers *Cupressus arizonica* toxic. It should not be used.

smoothing transitions, especially the loss of loved ones and the ending of relationships.

**Davana (*Artemisia pallens*)**

*Family:* Asteraceae

*Habitat & Growth:* Native to India. Annual herb grows to about 18 inches.

*Scent:* Fruity, blueberry, and sweet with moss tone (like the forest floor). The color is reddish-orange with a warm, amber hue.

*Components:* EO produced by one distiller near Mysore. S-D is from the plants cut before the flowers are open. Composition is cis-Davanone 75% ± and 10% Bicyclogermacrene and others.

*Properties, Indications, & Uses:* Mucolytic.

*Indicated for:* Coughing attacks with thick, ropelike mucus ("toux grasses et spasmodiques").

*Uses:* Often used in blends.

*Contraindications:* Not to be used on babies, children, and pregnant women. Considered a nerve toxin and abortive.

**Dill weed** and **seed (*Anethum graveolens*)**

*Family:* Apiaceae

*Habitat & Growth:* Annual herb native to the Mediterranean. Grows to a height of 4 feet.

*Scent:* Clear, spicy, herbaceous, grass, fresh, and clean. Warms the gut.

*Components:* Leaf and seed are S-D. Two oils are very different in composition. Seed oil mainly up to 60% Carvone which is much less present in the leaf oil.

*Properties, Indications, & Uses:* Mucolytic and anticatarrh.

*Indicated for:* Bronchial catarrh and insufficient liver function.

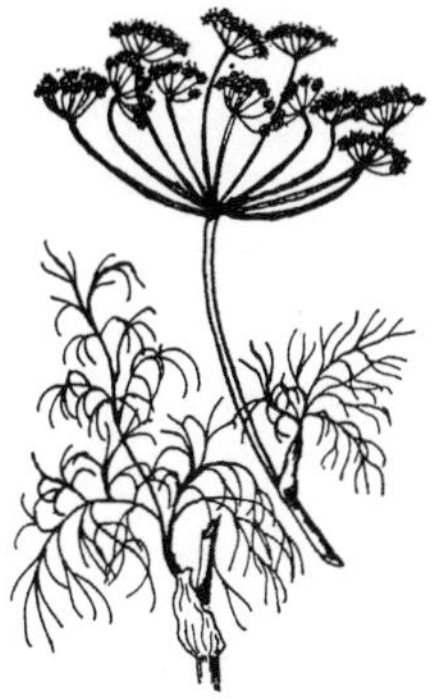

*Dill Weed*

*Uses:* Tea taken for flatulence of indigestion, for lack of menstruation, and to promote lactation. EO of seed and weed is much used in the commercial flavoring industry and is an excellent addition to culinary AT.

## Douglas Fir (*Pseudotsuga douglasii* also *P. menziesii*)

*Family:* Pinaceae

*Habitat & Growth:* Native to the West Coast of the United States. Now also grown elsewhere. A tall, attractive evergreen Fir tree much used in the Christmas tree industry.

*Scent:* Clear and fresh air conifer with a lemon-citrus note.

*Components:* S-D leaf oil; Components vary considerably. French oil contains large quantities of b-Pinene and smaller amounts of Citronellyl acetate and β-Phellandrene.

*Properties, Indications, & Uses:* Strongly antiseptic.

*Indicated for:* Respiratory infections.

*Uses:* Local disinfectant. This is one of the most lemon-scented of the Firs, with a powerful sweet and refreshing odor. Often used as a room freshener and scent in soap blends.

**Formula**

Mix 2 drams (1/4 oz.) Douglas Fir with 3 drops *Eucalyptus citriodora* or white grapefruit for a wonderful respiratory formula.

## Elecampane

See Inula.

## Elemi (*Canarium luzonicum*)

*Family:* Burseraceae

Gum Elemi is a soft, fragrant, and pathological exudation of a tree.

*Habitat & Growth:* Tree grows wild in the Philippine Islands.

*Scent:* Clear, soft, high, round, floral, fruity, and slightly herbaceous.

*Components:* Gum is S-D. Containing mainly d-a Phellandrene and Dipentene. With age the color turns darker and the optical rotation decreases which is similar to what happens to Angelica oil. It is assumed that color and optical rotation changes are due to the Phellandrene.

*Properties, Indications, & Uses:* Helps wounds to close.

*Indicated for:* Diarrhea, bronchitis, ulcers, and inhaled to treat thymus gland.

*Uses:* Cheap, easy to get, and suitable as a starting material to isolate Phellandrene in order to make synthetic oils.

**Eucalyptus**

*Family:* Myrtaceae

*Habitat & Growth:* Eucalyptus trees are tall, beautiful evergreen trees, up to 50 feet in height, and form 75% of the flora of Australia. They have also naturalized themselves in many other countries. They are S-D, especially in France, for a particular CT. They are sometimes called Gum Trees, but it is not the bark exudation that is S-D, rather the leaves. Eucalyptus globulus was discovered in Tasmania in 1792 and many names have been given to this tree. The botanical nomenclature is confusing, to say the least. *E. dives* is a species of Eucalyptus that can form *morphologically distinct forms*, even in close proximity to one another. One tree may produce an EO rich in Cineol, and other trees may produce an EO rich in another component. There are several forms of each Eucalyptus. Cineol was originally called Eucalyptol, is the principal constituent of the Eucalyptus oils, and has been prepared and used pharmaceutically since its discovery. Commercial Eucalyptol is 98% Cineol, is now a regular part of commerce, and is prepared from various forms of the Eucalyptus trees.

When Eucalyptus trees reach 3 to 4 years old, the tops are cut off to force the branches out. This is repeated for 7 to 8 years so that the trunk is large and has low, well-developed branches that are easy to cut. The leaves are harvested twice a year. Whole branches are cut off and the leaves and small twigs are removed and put into the distillery. Well-cultivated trees will form bushes that can yield 100 pounds of leaves per year. One acre can produce up to 35 thousand pounds of leaf material. On the average the leaves will produce up to 2% oil, so 35,000 pounds of leaf yields up to 350 kilos of oil.

*Scent:* Generally this group is camphoraceous, airy, and heady with woody subnotes. Eucalyptus species are include green, citrus, and peppermint.

*Properties, Indications, & Uses* of a variety of the Eucalyptus oils:

***E. polybractea.*** Common name is Blue Mallee. 70–90% Cineol among other components. Cineol form considered an expecto-

rant. *E. cryptonifera* form which contains 40% Cryptone and 10% Cineol is a mucolytic, antiviral, and antimalarial.
*Indicated for:* Malaria, chlamydia, various uterine problems, epididymitis, male sexual problems, and parasites of the gut.
***E. australiana.*** Contains 75% Cineol. Inhalant to cleanse the lungs. In great use medicinally.
***E. dives.*** Peppermint Eucalyptus. Contains 30% Phellandrene, up to 50% Piperitone, is a mucolytic.
*Indicated for:* A peppermint scented EO is inhaled for the sinuses and bronchials. Also applied for vaginal leucorrhea. Considered a slight neurotoxin and abortive. *E. dives* resembles *E. australiana* and is often substituted for it.
***E. citriodora.*** Lemon Eucalyptus. Much sought after as a construction tree. A high content of Citronellal. Aside from a high amount of Citronellal, it produces up to 20% Citronellol, which is more than Citronella grass. For this reason it is used in bug repellant mixtures. Considered analgesic, calming, sedative, and antihypertensive.
*Used for:* Cystitis and in bug repellant blends.
***E. campanulata.*** Contains up to 98% Methylcinnamate. Antispasmodic indicated for colitis and gut spasms.
***E. globulus.*** Contains up to 75% Cineol, 12% a-Pinene, with strong anticatarrh and expectorant properties, antibacterial, and antifungal. It makes mucus watery. It is not possible to inhale just-from-the-still EO, as it contains isovalraldehyde. This smelly component could trigger a strong coughing reflex, so the EO is rectified (redistilled) before use, and then it has great use as an inhalant.
*Indicated for:* Colds, flu, infected sinuses, laryngitis, bronchitis, and bacterial inflammation of the skin.
***E. radiata.*** Up to 72% Cineol, 20% Monoterpenes. Strongly antiviral and expectorant.
*Indicated for:* The respiratory system from top to bottom. Especially useful for vaginitis, acne, and sinus infections.

## Evergreens

See the essay, "Evergreens" in Chapter 6 and the individual listings in this chapter: Pine, Fir, Spruce, Cypress, Juniper, Douglas Fir.

## Fennel (*Foeniculum vulgare*)

*Family:* Apiaceae

*Habitat & Growth:* Native to the Mediterranean. Cultivated worldwide. A biennial or perennial herb up to 6 feet. Very pretty with feathery leaves. Two varieties: one with an edible root and another in which the seed is steam distilled to produce the oil. Produces up to 800 pounds of seed per acre.

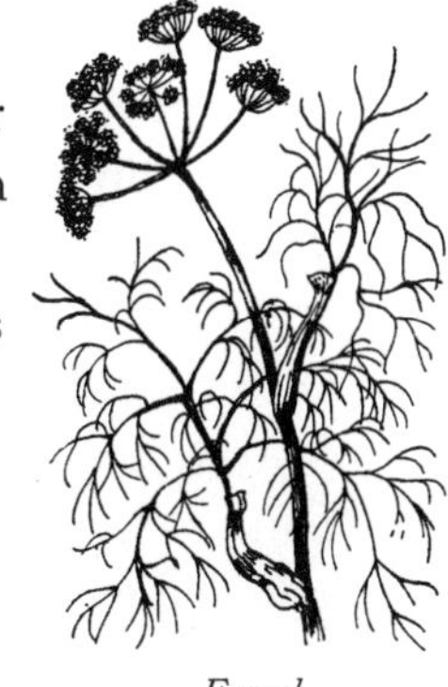
*Fennel*

*Scent:* Sweet, honey, licorice, and herbal notes. Pale, clear, gold oil.

*Components:* Varies widely. Seed oils are different from herb oils. Primarily δ-α–Pinene, Anethole up to 60% and Fenchone up to 22%, etc.

*Properties, Indications, & Uses:* The herb tea is a mild carminative and is used as a tonic aperitif tea and an emmenogogue. It also has psychoactive properties.

*Indicated for:* All types of stomach and intestinal disorders, breathing disorders of nervous origin, and pulmonary congestion. The estrogenlike EO is inhaled to help child birthing, to augment lactation, and is indicated for all types of menstrual problems from menarche to menopause.

*Uses:* The tea is very popular flavor in foods, breads, and pastries. The EO is a great addition in culinary AT.

## Fir

*Family:* Pinaceae

See Evergreen, Pine, Spruce, and Cedar. The Firs are distributed worldwide and are coniferous trees with pyramid shapes. EO generally S-D from small twigs and needles. A number of trees are called Fir.

*Abies ssp.*

*Tsuga canadensis,* Common Hemlock

*Tsuga heterophylla,* Prince Albert Fir or Western Hemlock

(See also Evergreen, Chapter 6)

*Pseudotsuga douglasii* or Douglas Fir. Covered under Douglas Fir.
*Pseudotsuga taxifolia.* See Evergreen, Chapter 6

Turpentine oil from *Pseudotsuga taxifolia.*

It is actually an oleo-resin produced in the crevices of the tree trunk. On S-D it produces up to 35% the volatile oil, which is composed of up to 55 % l-α-Pinene. Turpentine is used commercially in technical preparations. Turpentine oil is also produced from *Abies balsamea* (see below) called Canada Balsam Fir. This product is also a true turpentine because it consists of both resin and volatile oil. Component is principally l-α-Pinene.

***Abies siberica.*** Balsam Fir, grown widely in Russia. Chief constituent, 40% is l-Bornyl acetate. Properties are antispasmodic and used for bronchitis and asthma.

***Abies alba.*** White Fir. 95% Monoterpenes. Antiseptic. Inhaled for respiratory problems. In addition, *Abies alba* produces a cone oil with a very pleasant balsamic odor consisting chiefly of l-Limonene and used as an adjunct in many "Pine" needle scents.

***Abies balsamea.*** Balsam Fir. Up to 90% Monoterpenes. Properties are antiseptic and antispasmodic. Inhaled for the respiratory system.

***Abies sachalinensis, Abies mariana.*** These are called "Pine" needle oils, but are actually Firs. Commonly called Japanese Pine Needle. They contain mainly l-Limonene and Sesquiterpenes. Primarily used for respiratory inhalations and for scenting of soap.

**Frankincense**, called oil of Olibanum *(Boswellia carterii)*
*Family:* Burseraceae

Olibanum is the Frankincense of the ancients.

*Habitat & Growth:* Small trees growing in Somaliland and Southeast Arabia. Bark of the tree contains gum-oleo resin reservoirs. Natives incise the bark causing an exudation which, after a time, congeals into yellowish tears and drops. This is the gum of the ancient world. Various qualities of this gum can be called either Frankincense or Olibanum. The best quality is employed in church or temple incense for spiritual healing. The lowest grade and the least expensive is the one most often used for distillation of essential oil, and this is generally called oil of Olibanum.

*Scent:* Expansive, clean, dry, woody, conifer, fruity, dry, pepper, and spicy odor. Pale, green-gold oil.

*Components:* Pinene; Phellandrene; mainly Monoterpene hydrocarbons among others. There is also a small quality of Verbenone.

*Properties, Indications, & Uses:* It is considered antitumor and a strong immuno-stimulant with antidepressive and expectorant qualities.

*Indicated for:* Asthma, bronchial catarrh, immune deficiencies, and nervous depression. Particular value in perfume blends of the Oriental style, because it rounds out and gives alluring tones that are particularly difficult to identify as to the source. It has powerful value in the perfume and incense industry as a fixative as well as a main scent.

*Uses:* Has been used for 5000 years for spiritual healing and was used in ancient Egypt in the embalming process.

## Galanga (*Alpinia officinarum*)

*Family:* Zingiberaceae

*Habitat & Growth:* True Galanga is grown in Southeastern China. It is a reedlike plant about 3 feet tall and whose rhizomes are used in the spice trade and the EO industry. Similar species are True Ginger and Large Galanga (The dried rhizomes of *Alpinia galanga* is known as Large Galanga, and it is rarely available. Composition was mainly Cineol.)

*Scent:* Spicy and pepper.

*Components:* EO is extracted by SD from the gum. Pinene; Cadenene; and Sesquiterpenes among others.

*Properties, Indications, & Uses:* Antiseptic and disinfectant.

*Uses:* Certain types of flavors and perfumes.

## Galbanum (*Ferula spp.* often called *F. gummosa*)

*Family:* Apiaceae

Galbanum is produced as an excretion from the bases of the shoots and leaves. There are two types: soft and hard. Galbanum is one of those herbs that has been in use many thousands of years. The Romans considered it to be "the smell of green."

*Habitat & Growth:* Native to the Middle East. Large perennial herb with resinous ducts containing the exudation.

*Scent:* Weed, green and fatty odor with a bit of fruit. Clear to deep gold oil.

*Components:* Pinene; Cadinene; about 75% Monoterpenes.

*Properties, Indications, & Uses:* Tonic stimulant, anti-infectious, and powerfully resolves old emotional or spiritual problems.

*Indicated for:* All menstrual problems and for old skin lesions.

*Uses:* In previous years it was used as a stimulant inhalant, antispasmodic, and expectorant. The scent of Galbanum is something like Rose Geranium in that it is very specific. Once you have smelled either you will never forget them—and with Galbanum you will either like it or dislike it. Two to three drops in an 8 oz. blend is enough to fix the scent and bring a deep earthiness.

## Gardenia (*Gardenia augusta* or *G. florida* or *G. jasminoides* [Cape Jasmine])

*Family:* Rubiaceae

Gardenias are tropical and warm-weather flowers that have been used to scent tea as well as for some minor medicinal uses. The Chinese have a long history of using Gardenia *fruit* to treat vomiting of blood and for sores and boils, Gardenia *seeds* to treat rheumatism and twisted muscles, and *flowers* Gardenia and *roots* in tea form to regulate flow of blood and increase menstrual blood. There is **no** essential oil produced from Gardenia, and even if you see it in a catalog, it is in no way a natural (that is, produced from a plant) product. Gardenia scent is not produced by enfleurage. The only source for the scent of Gardenia that I am aware was once the oil produced by an aromatherapist by the continuous infusing and macerating of large quantities of fresh Gardenia blossoms in oil. The fragrant infused oil that is produced is a wonderful addition to massage oil blends or body lotions and has some history as a powerful aphrodisiac. Try it yourself, if you have quantities of Gardenia available.

*Scent:* A combination of Jasmine, Massoïa, and some Ylang-Ylang.

## Garlic (*Allium sativum*)

*Family:* Liliaceae

*Habitat & Growth:* Called "The Stinking Rose," it is thought to have originated in Siberia. This strongly scented perennial herb can grow up to 4 feet with a fat, underground bulb made up of several parts called cloves.

*Scent:* Strong, funky, pungent, powerful odor.

*Components:* S-D from fresh bulbs. Diallyl disulfides.

*Properties, Indications, & Uses:* Powerful antibacterial, vermifuge with thyroid stimulant, and possible cortisonelike properties. Bulb is eaten to kill internal parasites and for other intestinal difficulties; during the eating, the allicin disperses throughout the body via the blood stream, disinfecting wherever it goes, to finally cleanse the respiratory system upon the exhaled breath. It is also a mucolytic.

*Uses:* The EO can be used in extremely small quantities, diluted for inhalation or ingestion. Garlic has been in use since antiquity as a prophylactic and curative of all sorts of intestinal and respiratory ailments. Phoenician sailors carried large amounts of Garlic on their voyages. People of the world have complained since time immemorial of "garlic breath." It's even in Egyptian wall writings. For cosmetic and therapeutic use, see all Jeanne Rose writings.

**Caution:** Do not use pure EO of Garlic in the auditory canal, use only *infused* oil of Garlic.

## Geranium (*Pelargonium graveolens* or *P. x asperum*)

(This oil should be called Pelargonium oil.)

*Family:* Geraniaceae

See also Zdravetz, Geranium oil

There is much confusion in the names of oils called *Geranium* and Rose Geranium *(Pelargonium spp.)*. The Rose Geranium EO certainly does not come from the genus of plants *Geranium*, which produce mainly an astringent root, the tea of which is used for excessive blood loss such as hemorrhoids or menorrhagia and for tightening the vaginal opening. There is great controversy as to which constitutes Geranium EO and Rose Geranium EO, as the *Pelargoniums* readily cross and hybridize. The name

Geranium is used for both *Pelargonium* oil and Geranium oil and is used interchangeably.

I believe that Rose Geranium EO is derived from any number of cultivars of *Pelargonium* possessing a large amount of Geraniol and that so called Geranium EO is a Pelargonium possessing mostly Citronellol.

*Habitat & Growth:* The *Pelargoniums* grow wild in Cape Province, South Africa, and have been exported to the rest of the world where they are grown extensively for their fragrant leaves. It is a perennial shrub up to 5 feet with hairy leaves of various sizes and shapes.

*Scent:* Herbaceous, green, floral, sweet, and dry odor; it affects the first chakra. Color is a golden-brown to emerald-green.

*Components:* The EO is S-D. There are over 700 cultivars of *Pelargoniums,* all of which are called Geranium. Monoterpenes, with Geraniol with varied amounts of other components making up the chemotypes Menthol, Linaloöl.

*Properties, Indications, & Uses:* Mild antibacterial, mild antifungal, very good tonic astringent for the skin, hemostatic, and mild pancreas stimulant. Inhaled as a relaxant and anti-inflammatory.

*Indicated for:* All conditions of the woman's reproductive system as an inhalant and massage application. Indicated as well for all problems of the nervous system such as anxiety, agitation, and nervous fatigue. This is one of our most useful essential oils in perfumes, inhalations, and applications.

*Uses:* To stimulate the healthy output of adrenocortical glands and for menopause.

The parent plant of all *Pelargonium* varieties in commerce is *P. graveolens*. Most often produced commercially in 'Geranium' *(Pelargonium)* plantations in Grasse, France, and then exported from there. Easily propagated by cuttings. S-D comes from everything above ground, particularly the leaves or the top third of the plant in flower.

**Réunion 'Geranium' oil.** Most of the world's supply comes from this area, formerly called Bourbon which is an island east of Madagascar. Very strong roselike odor with a high Citronellol content and golden color.

**Madagascar 'Geranium' oil.** Most of this product is shipped to France. The scent is not as strong as the Réunion oil.

**Algerian 'Geranium' oil (African Geranium oil).** Possesses a strong, roselike odor not as delicate as that of the French oil, But more refined than the Réunion oil.

**Réunion oil**—Geraniol 50% and Citronellol 50%.

**Algerian oil**—Geraniol 80% and Citronellol 20%

**Spanish oil**—Geraniol 65% and Citronellol 35%

**Moroccan 'Geranium' oil.** Golden in color. Has an exceptionally high Citronellol content and about 67% Geraniol.

**Concrète and absolute of 'Geranium.'** Concrète is a waxy, dark green, solid mass only partly soluble in alcohol. Absolute is liquid, green, and totally soluble in alcohol. Both have a fine, soft Geranium odor. A fine addition when you wish to have green color in the resultant blends and perfumes.

**French 'Geranium' oil.** Possesses a fine, delicate roselike odor.

**Spanish 'Geranium' oil.** Produced in very small quantities. Is esteemed for its fine rose odor.

**Italian 'Geranium' oil.** Probably produced in Sicily and Calabria. Produced from ***Pelargonium roseum.***

**Egyptian 'Geranium' oil.** Has a remarkably high Citronellol content with outstanding uses in soaps and cosmetic preparation.

**Congo 'Geranium' oil.** Up to 44% Citronellol not readily available at this time.

**North American 'Geranium' oil.** Production is hampered by the high cost of American workers since most of the harvesting is done by hand. Not yet an important part of the trade, although its production for hydrosol is on the rise. 'Geranium' hydrosol is used for a variety of aromatherapy applications from a spritz to soothe hot flashes, to an ingredient in body care products. The North American 'Geranium' is preferable because hydrosols are perishable and often imported hydrosols are spoiled while hydrosols grown and distilled domestically are more likely to be fresh.

**Russian 'Geranium' oil.** Cultivated but not often exported since the Chernobyl nuclear disaster; it is probably now growing on nuclear contaminated soils. Not recommended for use, although some perfume companies have suggested this as a good crop to be exported to other parts of the world to provide employment to the people of the Chernobyl area.

**East African 'Geranium' oil.** Probably from *P. graveolens* (called Mawah oil) with two types: one high in Geraniol and Menthone and low in Citronellol, and the other high in Citronellol with no Geraniol.

There are numerous varieties of other *Pelargoniums* from various parts of Africa (where it is indigenous), which have not yet been well developed.

***Geranium macrorrhizum* oil (Bulgarian Geranium oil)** called Zdravetz oil.

This oil is from *Geranium macrorrhizum* and is incorrectly called Herb Robert. The volatile oil is S-D from the over-ground parts of the plant, and the odor is somewhat like Clary Sage, Orris, and Rose. It is often used to adulterate Bulgarian Rose oil. See Zdravetz.

## Ginger (*Zingiber officinale*)

*Family:* Zingiberaceae

One of the most important and oldest of spices.

*Habitat & Growth:* Native to Asia. Extensively cultivated throughout the tropics. It is an erect perennial herb, up to 3 or 4 feet, possessing a tuberous, thick, spreading rhizome (root) which is very strongly fragrant, up to 3% EO.

*Scent:* Hot, spicy, earthy, and woody, or hot, spicy, and sweet. Golden colored oil.

*Components:* EO prepared by S-D from the sun dried rhizomes, called "hands." Ginger components most of which are Sesquiterpenes; Linaloöl; Phellandrene among others.

*Properties, Indications, & Uses:* Powerful tonic for the entire digestive system. Sometimes considered an aphrodisiac.

*Indicated for:* Problems of the appetite and gut spasms.

*Uses:* To combat jet lag and motion sickness. The herb and the oil are one of the most used products in the flavor industry. For a tonic digestive, try one drop of Ginger EO mixed in a glass of commercial ginger ale. This is a delicious and helpful drink if you are having a stomachache after a large meal. This could also be considered a digestive bitter. Another Ginger is sometimes mentioned *(Zingiber cassumunar)*. This one in particular is used by inhalation as an anti-inflammatory and bronchodilator, indicated for all types of bronchitis and asthma.

The oleo-resin Ginger is also produced. As with Black Pepper, the EO derived by S-D of Ginger represents only the aromatic parts of the spice; it does not contain the non-volatile, pungent taste principles for which Ginger is appreciated. To obtain both the pungency and the fragrance, ground Ginger is cooked with volatile solvents to produce an oleo-resin. This contains Gingerol and Zingerone.

**Gotu Kola (*Centella asiatica*)** Common name is Indian Pennywort

*Family:* Apiaceae

*Habitat & Growth:* This is a small perennial herb distributed widely. Green, strongly odiferous EO.

*Scent:* Strong, brown, nutty.

*Components:* S-D. Camphor, Cineol, N-Dodecane, an unidentified Terpene that totals 36% of the EO, also Farnesene, etc.

*Properties, Indications, & Uses:* This herb is available as a powdered extract that can be reconstituted in liquid. It is used for all manner of serious skin conditions and has powerful uses for the skin care industry. It is antiinflammatory, soothing, and healing. It is also available from one company as a thick dark oil (the herb infused in oil?). This oil can be substituted for the oil in any formula.

*Indicated for:* Mind (leaf tea) and skin. The infused oil is used for serious skin diseases.

*Uses:* Serious skin diseases, even including leprosy and scleroderma. The EO is in use in United States cosmetic industry for skin problems. An infused oil is available from many companies for skin care.

**Grapefruit peel (*Citrus paradisi*)**

*Family:* Rutaceae

"Pamplemousse" in French.

*Habitat & Growth:* Native to Asia. Cultivated tree over 30 feet in height.

*Scent:* Citrus, floral, fruity, and aldelhyde odor. Clear to pink-yellow oil.

*Components:* EO cold-pressed from peel. 90% Limonene among many other components such as Citronellal.

*Properties, Indications, & Uses:* External astringent in formulations for oily skin or hair. Used internally in mixtures for the gall bladder.

*Indicated for:* Local disinfection of rooms; can be added to cleaning waters or sprayed.

*Uses:* Externally for cellulite. Inhaled for depression and headaches. Powerful uses for oily and congested skin. All over hair and body toner. The tea is used internally for obesity and water retention.

**Grapefruit seed** oil

See Citrus

**Guaiac Wood** (***Guaiacum officinale*** or from ***Bulnesia sarmienti***)

*Family:* Zygophyllaceae

*Habitat & Growth:* Native to South America. A wild, tropical tree up to 12 feet with a gnarled and crooked appearance.

*Scent:* Warm, fresh and smoky with a sweetish afternote.

*Components:* S-D from pieces of wood and sawdust. Up to 70% Guaiol which is a Sesquiterpene alcohol and other components.

*Properties, Indications, & Uses:* Stimulant and lymphatic decongestant.

*Indicated for:* Aesthenic, to decongest pelvic area. Usually used in massage blends.

*Uses:* Fragrance is complementary, such that it is used in Rose-type blends. Has lasting qualities and so is used as a natural fixative. Reasonably priced and much used in soaps and cosmetics.

**Helichrysum** (***Helichrysum angustifolium*** and other spp.)

*Family:* Asteraceae

This group of plants is commonly called Everlasting.

*Habitat & Growth:* Native to the Mediterranean. Cultivated elsewhere. Strongly scented herb up to 2 feet with bright, daisylike flowers. Called Everlasting because as the flowers dry, they retain color.

*Scent:* Strong honey and hay odor with herbaceous notes. Greenish colored oil.

*Components:* Entire above-ground plant is S-D to produce a sweet, honeylike, aromatic fragrance considered by some to be of Rose and Chamomile. Neryl acetate, Nerol, Pinene, and italidone. The concrète S-D for their EO. Many varieties of *Helichrysum* are S-D for the EO. Others include *Helichrysum stoechus*, and *H. italicum.*

*Properties, Indications, & Uses:* The French primarily use this as an anti-inflammatory to regulate cholesterol, stimulate the cells of the liver, and as an antispasmodic. Italian everlast has powerful antibruise properties.

*Indicated for:* Primarily indicated to resolve old scar tissue, for the Bartholin glands, and as an application for arthritis. Another interesting use is as a massage on the contracted penis and for Dupuytrens contracture (when the fingers contract into the palm). I personally have had great results applying Heliochrysum (in a 10% mixture) on my painful arthritic fingers.

*Uses:* Antiviral and regenerative, it stimulates the production of new cells, treats burns, scars, and acne. It is also detoxifying and can be used for drug (including cigarette) withdrawal.

## Heliotrope (*Heliotropium peruvianum*)

*Family:* Boraginaceae

Heliotrope is **not** processed for its fragrance. This plant is very fragrant usually with purple flowers that smell like cherry pie.

## Hemlock-Spruce

(See Spruce)

## Hinoki (*Chamaecyparis obtusa*) trunk, root, and needles.

(See Cypress)

## Honeysuckle (*Lonicera spp.*)

*Family:* Caprifoliaceae

*Habitat & Growth:* A perennial vine producing sweet-scented flowers.

*Scent:* Sweet, floral, honey, and fatty. Infused oil is golden.

*Components:* The flowers can be infused in oil to make an incredibly sweet-scented massage oil for all sorts of external conditions. NOT available as an absolute. Not much is known of the components.

**Formula**

Fill a clean, 1-quart mason jar with young flowers, then add olive oil until the jar is just full and just to the point where the flowers are submerged. Keep in a warm place, but not in the sun. Strain out the oil every 24–36 hours, and add new flowers to the oil until it takes on the scent of the flowers. Do not squeeze the flowers. Bottle in small containers, and refrigerate.

## Hops (*Humulus lupulus*)

*Family:* Moraceae

*Habitat & Growth:* Native to Europe. Perennial creeping, twining herb up to 12 feet. Bears scaly cones, called strobiles, containing a fragrant, granular powder called Lupulin. It is related to Marijuana, which is also processed for its essential oil.

*Scent:* Funky, musty, dirty, vegetative, and herbaceous. Very pale yellow color.

*Components:* EO by S-D from strobiles or cones. Very deep, rich odor. Humulene, other Sesquiterpenes, and over 100 other components.

*Properties, Indications, & Uses:* Estrogenlike, sedative, and antispasmodic.

*Indicated for:* Tachycardia, nervous gastritis, and insomnia.

*Uses:* Mostly in flavoring liquors and in some perfume blends. Has powerful use as a soporific. Used to reduce sexual overactivity.

*Contraindications:* Not for use on those who are hormone dependant.

## Horseradish (*Amoracia rusticana*)

*Family:* Brassicaceae (Cruciferae)

*Habitat & Growth:* Probably native to Eastern Europe. Now common throughout Russia, Europe, and Scandinavia. Perennial plant with leaves up to 50 cms. long. White flowers with a thick, whitish, tapering root that is easily propagated.

*Scent:* Very toxic and white-hot odor. Take extreme care when smelling.

*Components:* S-D from broken roots which have been soaked in water. Allyl isothiocyanate 75%; phenyllethyl isothiocyanate.

*Properties, Indications, & Uses:* Antibiotic, antiseptic, diuretic, carminative, expectorant, mild laxative, rubefacient, and stimulant.

*Uses:* Culinary preparations.

*Contraindications:* Oral toxin, dermal irritant, and mucous membrane irritant. Considered hazardous in essential oil form and not recommended for therapeutic or home use.

## Hyacinth (*Hyacinthus orientalis*)

*Family:* Liliaceae

*Habitat & Growth:* Native to Asia Minor and said to be of Syrian origin. Currently cultivated in Holland and Southern France. Most EO sold on market is synthetic. The absolute is available.

*Scent:* Absolute is floral, aldehyde, and strong.

*Components:* Concrète and absolute by solvent extraction of the flowers. EO from S-D of absolute. Phenylethyl alcohol, benzaldehyde, cinnamaldehyde, benzyl alcohol, benzoic acid, benzyl acetate, benzyl benzoate, eugenol, methyl eugenol, and hydroquinone, among others.

*Properties, Indications, & Uses:* Antiseptic, balsamic, hypnotic, sedative, and styptic properties. Indicated for the nervous system, stress, mental fatigue, and developing the creative side of the brain.

*Uses:* Often used in perfumery. Sweet, floral fragrance blends well with Narcissus, Violet, Ylang-Ylang, Styrax, Galbanum, Jasmine, and Neroli.

## Hyssop (*Hyssopus officinalis*)

*Family:* Lamiaceae

*Habitat & Growth:* Perennial shrub native to Southern Europe. Naturalized in the United States.

*Scent:* Herbaceous and vegetative with slightly meaty note, but fresh.

*Components:* Leaves and tops contain EO extracted by S-D. Pinene + almost 50% Pinocamphone as well as Sesquiterpenes.

*Properties, Indications, & Uses:* Two varieties are mentioned in Franchomme and Pénoël's *L'aromatherapie:*

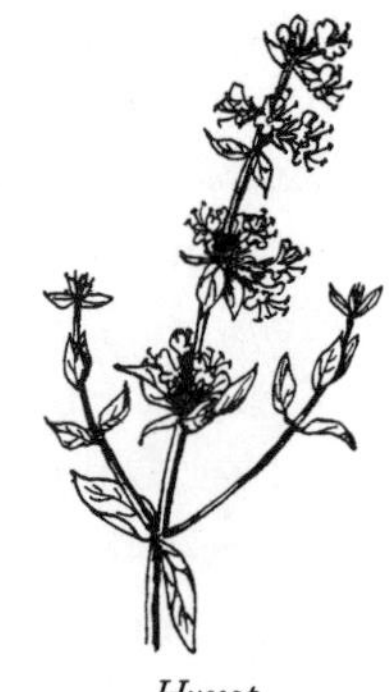
*Hyssop*

*H.O.* var. *decumbens* used as a potent viricide with an action against strep bacteria and bacterias in the naso-pharynx and tonsillitis. Tonic stimulant. Very therapeutic on sinusitis, bronchitis, and all aspects of the respiratory system. Inhaled for nervous depression.

*H.O. ssp. officinalis.* Strong anticatarrh, anti-asthmatic, and anti-inflammatory on the pulmonary system. Ability to regulate fat metabolism. Viricide.
*Indicated for:* Pneumonia, conditions of the nose and throat, and troubles of the ovaries, especially at puberty. A drop in a glass of warm water or vinegar and gargled is a powerful adjunct against tonsillitis. Plant used as an aromatic in liquors, tonics, and bitters.
*Contraindications:* Not to be used on children and pregnant women. This subspecies is considered neurotoxic and abortive.

## Immortelle

(See Helichrysum)

## Inula (*Inula spp.*)

*Family:* Asteraceae

Several species of Inula are used in AT work.

Elecampane from *I. helenium.* Plant is a coarse perennial native to Asia. Cultivated in many places. The root has internal parasite killing properties. The greatest part of the S-D EO Alantolactone. This is a mucolytic, antifungal, and anthelminthique. Used for purulent bronchitis with much expulsion of mucus. Root tea mixed with Black tea creates a potent antiasthmatic (bronchodilating) therapeutic tea.

*I. graveolens* Common name is Inula odora. Properties are heart regulatory and powerful mucolytic. One of the most powerful essential oils to be used in respiratory crisis. Inula can be considered shock therapy for the respiratory system and can be used in a diffuser over a long period of time to disinfect and heal an infected ear, nose, or throat.

*Indicated for:* Arrythmia and conditions of the ear, nose, throat, and tonsils. External use for treating skin rashes, eruptions, and herpes.

## Iris

See Orris root.

The Iris flowers are rarely, if ever, used in commercial perfumery but can be used by the home distiller or maker of infused massage products.

## Jasmine (*Jasminum officinale* [French Jasmine], *J.o. var. grandiflorum* [Spanish Jasmine] and *J. sambac* [Tea Jasmine])

*Family:* Oleaceae

As people in the perfume and AT are wont to say, "This is the King of Flowers."

*Habitat & Growth:* There are many species of Jasmine. It is thought to be native to China, but is now cultivated worldwide. Jasmine is either an evergreen shrub or a vine that can climb up to 30 feet high and wide.

*Scent:* The leaves are bright green, and the beautiful white flowers are very fragrant with its very specific scent. Intensely floral and fatty with musk or civet notes and some hay and honey.

*Components:* Jasmine is a classic example of a flower that continues to develop and emit its natural odor up to 24 to 36 hours after it has been picked; therefore, it is supremely suitable for the enfleurage technique of extracting the scent via maceration in warm fat. A concrète and absolute are obtained by petroleum ether and high-proof alcohol. The concrète is reddish-brown and waxy with a powerful odor. The absolute is clear yellowish-brown with a beautiful odor more characteristic of the live flowers. On steam or water distillation, Jasmine flowers give a low yield of oil, but the hydrosol may be useful.

Process of enfleurage was developed in Southern France in the eighteenth century and is wonderfully discussed in the book

*Perfume* by Patrick Suskind.[3] The how-to of this process is discussed in *The Aromatherapy Book: Applications & Inhalations* by Jeanne Rose and can be easily employed by the home perfumer to make wonderful essences of Jasmine, Lily, Lilac, and other thick-petalled flowers. Enfleurage is a highly labor-intensive work. An absolute of the chassis of enfleurage can be obtained, and this process is used by high-quality perfumers in France. You may read about this in *The Essential Oils, vol. I* by Ernest Guenther, page 333.

Over 100 components including Lactones such as Jasmone, Linaloöl, Geraniol, and Nerol. The Lactones give the scent a powerful, deep, earthy, lasting, almost fruitlike odor. Benzyl acetate 65%, Linaloöl 15%, Linalyl acetate 8%, Benzyl alcohol 6%, Jasmone 3%, Indole 3%.

Indole is a natural constituent of the flowers of Spanish Jasmine. As soon as the flower buds open in the morning, the Indole is freed and evaporates into the atmosphere. Toward evening, when the flowers close, the Indole disappears back into the tissues of the plant to reappear again the following morning at daybreak; therefore, the ideal time to handpick Jasmine flowers is at daybreak, when the flowers are the most fragrant and have the highest percentage of components intact.

*Uses:* Indispensable in perfumes and is used in the finest and most well-known perfumes; hardly a perfume is conceived without a bit of Jasmine in its blend to add a smoothness and elegance. Used in cosmetics and facial preparations for dry, greasy, irritated, and sensitive skin. Of great value is a drop applied to the temples to relieve headache. Wonderful as a massage for the pelvic area for a congested pelvis or for any type of menstrual problems. Used to balance women's hormones to create a regular menstrual cycle. Inhaled, it can be a great help for labor pains, and applied externally, it is a massage for the uterus. Used to obviate depression, relieve nervous exhaustion, and ease stress from any type of circumstance. It can make one feel happy and joyful and, to this end, is a great substitute if Spearmint oil does not work. One species of Jasmine is used to scent black tea, this is the Jasmine sambac.

---

[3]Patrick Suskind. *Perfume.* NY, NY Pocket Book, 1985..

Jasmine is one of the most expensive AT products, and because it is not S-D, some do not consider it an AT product; in any case, it can cost $4000 a kilo and up.

There are three very specific scents to Jasmine: One is very fruity and sweet; another is a powerful, deep odor with hints of scatol; and another with a somewhat more typical household Jasmine odor. Also, these oils range from a deep, golden, yellow brown to brown. I have heard aromatherapy teachers dismiss the rankish scatol odor as atypical of Jasmine and determine it to be "synthetic and dilute." I find this behavior on the part of our AT teachers reprehensible. There are very few of us with the "nose" to be able to pick up an absolute and dismiss it as pure and/or synthetic out of hand. If a teacher does this to you, dismiss them as having poor ethics and question their motives.

## Juniper berry (*Juniperus communus*)

*Family:* Cupressaceae

*Habitat & Growth:* The common Juniper is a native to the Northern Hemisphere. Evergreen shrub or tree up to 18 feet. Has narrow, stiff, prickly needles and little brown berries that turn black in the second or third year.

*Scent:* Coniferous, woody, spicy, and herbal odor. A clear oil.

*Components:* S-D of berries. Very rich, deep aroma. 8% resins; 0.4% Juniperene; Pinene and Terpinenes.

*Properties, Indications, & Uses:* Expectorant and antiseptic.

*Indicated for:* Bronchitis and externally for rheumatism.

**Junipers** include:

Berry oil of subspecies *J. terpineoliferum* which is rich in Terpineols and is used as a dissolver of kidney stones and as a tonic for the digestive system and pancreas.

*Indicated for:* All sorts of treatments for the pancreas and kidney. The EO from the wood of *J. mexicana* ("Cedarwood") is used for hemorrhoids and to decongest the veinal system.

The EO from the stems of *J. sabina* are used as an external application for rheumatism. Not recommended for internal use.

The EO from the wood of *J. virginiana* ("Cedarwood") is indicated for hemorrhoids, the hydrosol as an antibacterial cleaner for the home.

*Juniperus procera* (East African Cedarwood)

*Juniperus oxycedrus* the berry, leaf, and wood are S-D to produce three different EO. The wood oil is generally called oil of Cade (See Cade). It is an empyreumatic wood oil that is also commonly called oil of Juniper tar and often used in medicinal products for dandruff or scales on the skin such as eczema.

*Juniperus sabina* (Savin) is an ancient plant that when distilled contains mainly Sabinol. It has had much use as an antirheumatic, vermifuge, and emmenogogue, but is very toxic and has had irritating side effects. Not recommended for use.

**Kewda (*Pandanus odoratissimus*)** Hawaiian name **Hala.**

*Family:* Pandanaceae

*Habitat & Growth:* "This tree is well known in Hawaii. It is rugged and grows very high, its branches spreading far apart in all directions. The leaves are long, and lined with sharp spikes. The leaves are used in hat- and matmaking. The trunk rests on tubular roots, far above the ground. The flowers come in large clusters enveloped with long, white, and very fragrant leaves. The fruit is made up of a large number of small bodies containing its seed, also comes in cluster form. The small bodies are very fragrant and because of this they are frequently called flowers..."[4]

This is the family of Screw-pines often used in basketry and hatmaking. The seeds are dispersed by the sea, fresh water, turtles, fish, birds, and bats.

*Scent:* Kewda is the essential oil that has a powerful odor reminiscent of Gardenia and Horseradish. Even so, the scent is sweet, powerful, and appealing. This plant is particularly cultivated for its scent which comes from the male flowers.

*Components:* A difficult oil to examine, one sample I have seen had 64% beta-phenylethyl methyl ether, 16% Terpinene-4-ol, 5% gamma-Terpinene. This is considered a novel oil.

*Properties, Indications, & Uses:* Perfumery.

[4] *Hawaiian Herbs of Medicinal Value,* trans. by Akaiko Akana, from the compilation of Messrs. Kaaia Kamanu and J. K. Akina. Pacific Book House, Honolulu, Hawaii. 1922.

*Uses:* The *flower* is chewed and the juice is taken for constipation, the dose is 16 flowers per dose. The *root* is used for birthing problems or for chest pain. The plant is cultivated for its ornamental value and is a staple on some Pacific atolls where a black dye is prepared from the *roots*. The oil is used in perfumery for a very particular note.

**Perfume Fixatives**

| **Animal Fixatives** | **Vegetable Substitutes** |
|---|---|
| Ambergris-whale | Labdanum |
| Civet-cat | Spikenard |
| Castorium-beaver | Galbanum/Oakmoss/Carrot seed |
| Musk-deer | Musk-ambrette/Cistus |
| | Oakmoss |
| | Opopanax |

## Labdanum (*Cistus ladanifer*)

*Family:* Cistaceae

*Habitat & Growth:* Perennial shrub up to 6 feet. Grows wild, in large stands, and in warm sheltered places on some Mediterranean islands.

*Scent:* Fragrant and unforgettable balsamic odor of musk and smoke.

*Components:* There are five products produced (For more description, see Guenther, Vol. VI, p. 46):

1. Crude gum. It is prepared by boiling the dried leaves and twigs in water. It is then skimmed off the surface of the water and dried. Crude gum smells very much like ambergris and is a vegetable substitute for this mammalian product. See table that follows.
2. Resinoid of Labdanum. The crude gum is treated with alcohol and filtered.
3. Oil of Labdanum. EO prepared by S-D of the crude gum. This is the most valuable of the perfumer's raw materials. It is sometimes marketed as a synthetic ambergris.
4. The concrète and absolute of Labdanum. Prepared by extract-

*An Animal Fixative*

The musk deer *Moschus Moschiferus Family:* Cervidae (she xiang) is distributed in Tibet, Northern India, and Siberia. The part used in the past and today in some very high end and expensive perfumes is the dried secretion of the preputial follicles. The Chinese consider the nature of this product to be pungent and warm, to have an affinity for the heart and the spleen, and to have a resuscitative effect, as well as being cardiotonic, promoting circulation, and acting as a stimulant.

*Indicated for:* Fainting, delirium, semiconscious states, traumatic injuries, amenorrhea, and retained placenta or fetus.

*Contraindications:* It is considered an abortive for pregnant women. The usual dose is 0.2–0.4 g. This animal is endangered, and the product should not be used by the informed consumer.

Since 1968, when I first began to collect essential oils and flower scents obtained by enfleurage, I have also made a collection of vegetable and animal fixatives, including all of those mentioned in the above chart. This library of ancient scents proves that some odors definitely improve with age. In particular the animal odors, although some of the vegetable fixatives have also thickened and improved with age.

ing the dried twigs and leaves with solvents. It is used in cosmetics, perfumes, and soaps, as a warm balsamic tone in perfume blends, and as an excellent natural fixative.

5. Oil of Labdanum. The EO by S-D of the dried and fresh leaves and twigs. This oil produces a terpenelike odor different from the plant exudation and is of little use.

Composition includes Terpenes, Acetophenone, and other Ketones, etc.

*Properties, Indications, & Uses:* Antiviral, antibacterial, and antiarthritic.

*Indicated for:* Children's illnesses, whooping cough, and inflammation of the arteries.

*Uses:* Skin care for mature skin and wrinkles and an inhalant for coughs and bronchitis. As a powerful fixative in perfumery to replace ambergris.

*Other uses:* Labdanum has a powerful ability to bring up past lives and past or buried memories. Very helpful in ritual work.

**Lanyana (*Artemisia afra*)** Common name is **African absinthe**
*Family:* Asteraceae
*Habitat & Growth:* Unknown.
*Scent:* Warm and sharp.
*Components:* Alcohols; Terpenes; Ketones.
*Properties, Indications, & Uses:* Mucolytic and vermicide.
*Indicated for:* Migraine headaches and problems of the bronchial and pulmonary system
*Contraindications:* Not to be used on babies, children, and pregnant women. Neurotoxin and abortive.

**Lavender (*Lavandula angustifolia*)**
*Family:* Lamiaceae
*Scent:* Powdery, floral, light, and clean A pale yellow oil.
*Components:* Mainly Linalyl acetate and Linaloöl with additions of Geraniol.

This is the oil that is often adulterated, but this is the one that is the most desired for therapy.

*Properties, Indications, & Uses:* Calming. Few negative qualities. Sedative, muscular relaxant, anti-inflammatory, and powerful tonic for entire system. Externally for skin conditions such as acne, to soothe burns and scalds, for hair and skin care; inhaled to ease depression, nervous tension and for relaxation; used in the birthing room with a diffusor during childbirth; has many diverse and soothing uses.

*Indicated for:* Hiccups, insomnia, nervous conditions, and all types of skin conditions from childhood to the aged. Ulcers, cramps, etc. Inhaled for asthma and bronchitis. Restorative and tonic. Great in baths and all types of cosmetic products especially those used by men.

**Lavandin** ***(Lavandula x intermedia*** [a cross between ***L. angustifolia*** and ***L. latifolia***]***)***
*Scent:* Powdery, sweet, floral, and herbaceous smell. A pale yellow oil. If this oil is dark yellow it is of inferior quality with poor components.

*Components:* 45% Linaloöl, 25% Esters, 12% Aldehydes and Ketones. This oil was not available prior to 1930. Now it makes up most of what most people know as Lavender oil.

*Properties, Indications, & Uses:* Antibacterial and tonic to the nervous system.

*Indicated for:* Bronchitis, hypotensive, and for those suffering deep anguish.

*Uses:* Inhalant mixtures for the respiratory system. Has a sharper, more powerful scent than true Lavender and is good for the respiratory, muscular, and circulatory systems. The use for Lavandin can be the same as Lavender. In addition, Lavandin is taken internally in suppository form for a variety of respiratory conditions.

**Spike Lavender (*L. latifolia*)** aka **Aspic**

*Scent:* Camphoraceous, powdery, and herbaceous.

*Components:* Mainly Cineol and Camphor with Linaloöl and others.

*Properties, Indications, & Uses:* Mainly used for paralysis, rheumatism, and arthritis. Also has valuable expectorant and viricide properties.

*Indicated for:* Coughs, athlete's foot, and rhinitis.

**Spanish Lavender (*L. stoechas*)**

*Scent:* Camphoraceus, sharp, somewhat floral and herbaceous odor. Clear to yellow oil.

*Components:* Includes Camphor and Fenchone among others.

*Properties, Indications, & Uses:* Considered a powerful anti-infectious agent, especially for pseudomonas bacteria.

*Indicated for:* Earaches, eczema, and chronic sinusitis.

*Contraindicated:* Not to be used on babies and children.

## Lemon (*Citrus limon*)

*Family:* Rutaceae

*Habitat & Growth:* The origin of the Lemon tree is a mystery. It is a small, evergreen tree up to 20 feet. Although some consider it a native of Southeast China, others consider Lemon to be a sport or a hybrid of Citron and Lime. It is not mentioned in the early Roman writings, was unknown to the Romans, and apparently was introduced to the Middle East about A.D. 1100, as it was described in the Arabic herbals. Columbus introduced the Citrus fruits into the Americas in 1493. Seeds were planted in Haiti and the Dominican Republic and Citrus trees soon spread throughout the area. Lemons are primarily grown in the United States in California and are expressed for the EO in only some areas. On complete exhaustion by S-D, the peel from 2000 lbs. of Lemon fruit will yield 7 kg. ± of EO. Cold pressing yields less EO. Quality of the oil depends upon the region in which the Lemons are grown, just as in any other plant.

*Scent:* Clean, citrus, and sugary with a bit of spice.

**Italian Lemon oil** is produced in Sicily and Calabria. Often the color of this oil is a bit green. It was originally produced by hand-pressing (also called "sponge method"). Variation of quality depending on production location and weather variations. Also, the summer pressed oils have a lower Citral content than the winter oils. Italian Lemon oil often has constituents not observed in California Lemon oil.

**Lemon oil** is also produced Terpene free and Sesquiterpene free to produce an oil that is more soluble and more easily dissolved in alcohol. They are also less irritating.

*Components:* Primarily Limonene and Pinene with some Citral, Geraniol, and others.

**Spanish Lemon oil** was started in Malaga and other Spanish provinces in 1937.

**Palestine Lemon oil** began to be produced in the 1940s.

All of these oils mentioned have been of important use in the flavoring industry, especially in beverages, soft drinks, and baked goods. They also have great value in toiletries and impart a very refreshing top note.

One other Lemon oil deserves to be mentioned: oil of Petitgrain Lemon, which is Lemon leaf oil. This is formed from leaves and twigs, subjected to S-D, and provides a very bright, perky scent to any blend. The aromatic qualities of Lemon Petitgrain oil are due to the high proportion of Nerol. "It is a well-known fact that Nerol possesses, to a much higher degree than Geraniol, the property of communicating to the compounds in which it occurs, a peculiar pungency and tenacity."[5] There is a

[5] Ernest Guenther, *The Essential Oils,* Vol. III (Malabar, Fla: Kreiger Publishing) p. 118.

higher percentage of Nerol in Lemon Petitgrain than any other oil except for Neroli and Helichrysum.

***Citrus limon*** is antibacterial and antiseptic and has the ability to dissolve gallstones. The EO has some value in reducing the onset of nightmares.

*Indicated for:* Digestive and liver problems and to disinfect the air.

Lemon juice is a great addition to hot drinks for insomnia, colds, flus, and virus infections.

## Lemongrass (*Cymbopogon citratus*)

*Family:* Poaceae (Grass)

*Habitat & Growth:* Native to Asia. A tall, perennial grass that is very aromatic and grows up to 4 feet in height.

*Scent:* Citrus, herbaceous, and smoky.

*Components:* S-D from tops. Up to 85% Citral, up to 25% Myrcene.

*Properties, Indications, & Uses:* Tonic, digestive, and vasodilator with anti-inflammatory and sedative properties.

*Indicated for:* Promotion of good digestion and externally to massage out cellulite.

*Uses:* Excellent in skin care preparations, for athletes foot, excessive sweat, for scabies, as an insect repellant, and to tone all the tissues. One of the most important Eos, because Citral is the starting material for the preparation of many man-made aromatics.

## Lemon Petitgrain

(See Lemon)

## Lemon Verbena

(See Verbena)

## Lilac (*Syringa* spp.)

*Family:* Oleaceae

*Habitat & Growth:* Native to East Asia. Shrubs and small trees with showy flowers, usually strongly fragrant.

*Scent:* Fruity, floral, and aldehyde.

*Components:* Unknown.

*Properties, Indications, & Uses:* This does not exist in EO form. An Italian company says they hydrodiffuse the flowers with added synthetic ingredients to produce a delightful pink colored "EO." Most Lilac essential oil is synthetically made.

### Lime (*Citrus medica var. acida* aka *C. aurantifolia)*

*Family:* Rutaceae

There are a number of synonyms for Lime; please see Citrus.

*Habitat & Growth:* Small evergreen tree up to 12–15 feet Probably native to Asia. The sour fruit has a pale, green peel and is about the size of a small Lemon. There are a number of Limes: Florida, East Indian, Sweet Lime, Mexican, and others.

*Scent:* Citrus, tart, and sweet odor with some spice. Clear to greenish gold in color.

*Components:* Expressed for EO. Mainly Limonene, Pinenes.

*Properties, Indications, & Uses:* Used internally, it is antispasmodic. Juice is especially good for internal parasites.

*Uses:* Lime oil has extensive use in the body-care industry and forms, along with Lavender oil, a great deal of men's fragrances. Since Lime oil is so reasonably priced, it is often used in massage oils for its fresh fragrance.

### Linaloe (*Bursera spp.*)

*Family:* Burseraceae

*Habitat & Growth:* Primarily used is Linaloe from Mexico. EO distilled from wood and fruit. It is cheap and produces up to 50–80% Linaloöl; hence, it makes a great starting ground to extract Linaloöl for use in upgrading the Linaloöl content in other EOs. It may be where we get much of the Linaloöl for Lavender 40/42. I have not seen Linaloe available in any AT source list, but the French use it in their therapy as an antispasmodic for all spasmodic pathologies. Makes a great substitute for Rosewood.

*Scent:* Unknown.

### *Litsea cubeba* Common name is May Chang

*Family:* Lauraceae

*Habitat & Growth:* Native to East Asia. Cultivated in Asia. Small tropical tree with fragrant lemony-scented leaves. Small fruits are pepper shaped and from this shape comes the name *cubeba*. It is definitely not related to the Black Pepper plant, which is a vine, nor the Lemon Verbena shrub, which can be a tree.

*Scent:* Spicy, lemon, and citrus with vegetative notes.

*Components:* Up to 85% Citral. Often used as substitute for Lemon EO.

*Properties, Indications, & Uses:* Calming, sedative, and anti-inflammatory.

*Uses:* Inhaled for nervous depression and taken for gastric ulcers or poor appetite. In skin care it is used for acne and excessive oil. Also used as an insect repellant.

## Lovage (*Levisticum officinale*)

*Family:* Apiaceae

*Habitat & Growth:* Native to Southern Europe. Naturalized in North America. A tall perennial plant that looks like Celery. Grows to 6 feet in height. All parts of the plant contain volatile oil, although Lovage root oil is most important.

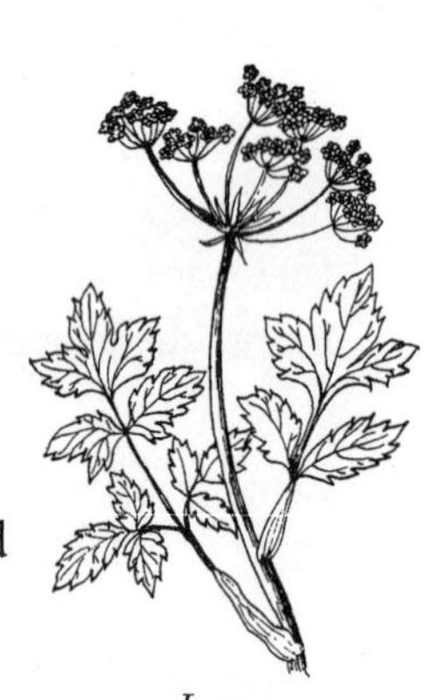

*Lovage*

*Scent:* Strong celery, vegetative, green, nutty, and caramel scent.

*Components:* EO S-D from both leaf and root. 70% Butylidene phthalides

*Properties, Indications, & Uses:* The French consider Lovage root and seed oil to have powerful antitoxic actions against poisons and as an antipsoriasis ingredient. Antiparasite effects, especially against tapeworm.

*Indicated for:* Serious digestive problems, psoriasis, weakness, and congestion of the liver.

*Uses:* As an ingredient in flavoring compositions such as tobacco, liquors, and food. Sometimes used in perfume blends for its particularly novel odor; however, it must be used very sparingly.

*Note:* I personally have never used Lovage oil except in demonstrations especially for its strong, green, celery odor.

## Macassar (*Schleichera oleosa*)

*Family:* Sapindaceae

An old plant whose seeds are S-D for the Bitter Almond odor

which was mixed with Olive oil to make a hair oil. The word "antimacassar" comes from the use of little lace doilies that were placed on the head of a chair to absorb this oil from the person's head so that the furniture would not be stained.

## **Mandarin** and **Tangerine** (***Citrus reticulata***)

*Family:* Rutaceae

There are two varieties of this oil. One called Mandarin, mainly from Europe, and the other called Tangerine, mainly from the United States. Some experts consider these plants to be the same, and some consider them to be either different varieties or different horticultural strains; however, the EO from both are used very much in the same manner.

*Habitat & Growth:* Native to southern China. Naturalized in many places. Small evergreen tree up to 20 feet with glossy leaves, fragrant flowers, and a sweet, fleshy fruit that is easy to peel.

*Scent:* Red mandarin is warm, citrus, fruity, and complex floral odor. Green mandarin has a marine note.

*Components:* Both oils contain mainly Limonene. Mandarin contains components not in Tangerine, such as methyl anthranilate, which is highly sedative. There is some difference in the scent and color, with Mandarin usually having a deeper, softer scent and a more deeply orange color.

*Properties, Indications, & Uses:* Relaxant, sedative, and hypnotic. *Indicated for:* Overexcited children, insomnia, and mental distress. *Uses:* One of the main uses for these EOs is as a soporific: one drop in a half a glass of hot water with honey makes a wonderful bedtime drink for children or sensitive adults.

## **Marjoram** (***Origanum majorana***)

*Family:* Lamiaceae

There is much confusion in regard to the Marjoram oils. The common name Marjoram can refer to any number of plants including some *Origanum spp.* and some *Thymus spp.* What we will discuss here is *Origanum majorana*.

*Habitat & Growth:* Native to the Mediterranean. A small, tender perennial up to 3 feet.

*Scent:* Warm, herbaceous, aldehyde, nutty, and woody.

*Components:* About 40% Terpenes among other components.

*Properties, Indications, & Uses:* Considered a powerful anti-aphrodisac. Strong antiseptic and mild diuretic with pain-relieving qualities.

*Indicated for:* Loss of muscle tone due to deadened nerves and problems with excessive thyroid function; cardiovascular disease; dyspnea; sexual difficulties, especially obsession with sex, excessive desire for sex, genital irritability or abnormal response to genital stimulation; psychic problems such as anxiety or stress; feelings of oppression; psychosis; insomnia; vertigo; and epileptic seizures.

*Use:* Externally for rheumatism and muscular aches and pains. Inhaled for respiratory infections. Ingested for digestive disturbances.

*Other uses:* A potent oil to inhale when there is pain or distress, especially if you mix it with Ylang-Ylang and also take a drop of Tangerine in honey. This is a very soothing and effective combination.

*Reminder*

There is much confusion with the Thymes, Marjorams, and Oreganos, and many retailers don't know the difference and will substitute one for the other. Some of these oils can be quite toxic and are contraindicated for all use, and some have no known toxicity. It is very important that the germinating aromatherapist pay attention to the differences in the color, feel, and "scentual" quality of these oils.

## Massoïa aka Massoy Bark (*Cryptocarya massoïa*)

*Family:* Lauraceae

*Habitat & Growth:* Grown in New Guinea and collected for centuries. Evergreen tree.

*Scent:* Fruity, coconut, hot, and tropical odor.

*Components:* Bark is S-D and $CO_2$ extracted. Containing mainly Lactones (which do not come over in the S-D).

*Properties, Indications, & Uses:* Anti-infectious and a major antibacterial.

*Indicated for:* Respiratory system from top to bottom and bacterial and fungus infections of the digestive system.

*Uses:* Medicinal value; forms an ingredient of Javanese medicines.

I personally like to use it, one drop per 8 servings, as an ingredient in Jasmine rice, added after the rice is cooked. The powerful Coconut odor in the rice is very appealing.
*Contraindications:* Not to be used on babies, children, and pregnant women. Powerful skin irritant if applied neat. Must be diluted before external use.

## Mastic (*Pistacia lentiscus*)

*Family:* Anacardiaceae
*Habitat & Growth:* Native to the Mediterranean. Mastic is produced mainly on the Greek island of Chios from the natural oleo-resin from the trunk of a small, bushy tree up to 10 feet.
*Scent:* Soft, warm and lightly fragrant.
*Components:* Mainly Pinenes.
*Properties, Indications, & Uses:* Mainly lymphatic decongestant.
*Indicated for:* Hemorrhoids, thrombosis, decongest the sinus, and inflammation of the prostate.
*Uses:* Mastic is the original Old World chewing gum. In Greece it is mixed with water and sugar to form a thick, white cream eaten by the spoonfuls as a sweetmeat with thick, bitter coffee or a strange Aromatherapy dinners.

## Melilot (*Melilotus officinalis*)

*Family:* Fabaceae
Common name is King's Clover or Sweet Hayflower
*Habitat & Growth:* Native to Europe and Asia. A bushy perennial herb up to 3 feet.
*Scent:* Hay and honey odor.
*Components:* Coumerins among others.
*Properties, Indications, & Uses:* Since the EO is not normally available, it has no use in AT; however, for the herbal use of this fragrant plant, see *The Aromatherapy Book: Applications & Inhalations* by Jeanne Rose or *Jeanne Rose's Herbal Body Book.*

## Melissa (*Melissa officinalis*)

*Family:* Lamiaceae
Common name is Balm or Lemon Balm
*Habitat & Growth:* Native to the Mediterranean. Naturalizes easily.

Reproduces by underground stems. An herbal plant up to 18 inches, spreading easily.

*Scent:* Citrus, herbaceous, vegetative odor with a bit of fern.

*Components:* S-D from tops and tender, green leaves, produces small quantity of oil, up to .02%. Mainly Geraniol, Linaloöl, with Citronellol and Citronellal.

*Properties, Indications, & Uses:* Hypotensive, hypnotic, and calming sedative with anti-inflammatory properties.

*Indicated for:* Insomnia, hysteria, nervous crisis, irritability, and great anger.

*Uses:* Herb tea taken internally for stomach cramps, indigestion, or nausea. A wonderful, fragrant oil that is often diluted with less expensive Lemon-scented oils. John Steele's chart on page 180–181 of *The Aromatherapy Book: Applications & Inhalations* by Jeanne Rose mentions Melissa oil several times, when in fact, it is Marjoram and Lemon that are actually used and should be listed.

### Mimosa absolute (*Acacia dealbata*)

*Family:* Mimosaceae

*Habitat & Growth:* Native to Australia. An attractive small tree up to 30 feet with fragrant flowers.

*Scent:* Honey, citrus, floral soft, and powdery smell. Deep yellow oil.

*Components:* Mainly available as an absolute or concrète. Mainly Hydrocarbons.

*Properties, Indications, & Uses:*

*Indicated for:* Old memories and stress.

*Uses:* Externally for sensitive or oily skin and skin problems caused by stress. Used by inhalation for nervous tension, sensitivity, and anxiety.

### Mint (*Mentha spp.*)

[Name used by Theophrastus, from the nymph Minthe.]

*Family:* Lamiaceae

About 30 species. Natives of the north temperate zone. The more or less characteristic odor of the species change during the progress of the life of the plant. Type species: *Mentha spicata* L. *Whorls of flowers in terminal spikes or some in the upper axis.* Plants glabrous or very nearly so, including *M. spicata, M. piperita, M.*

*citrata, M. longifolia, M. rotundifolia, M. alopecuroides, M. aquatica, M. cripsa.*

*Whorls of flowers all axillary*, including *M. cardiaca, M. arvensis, M. canadensis, M. gentilis.*

Mints include Pennyroyal, Peppermint, Japanese Mint (Menthol), Chinese Mint, Wild Mint, Brazilian Mint (Menthol), Spearmint, Watermint, and Bergamot Mint. I have covered Spearmint and Peppermint in alphabetical order with a discussion of Menthol under Mint, Corn Mint.

## Mint, Corn Mint (*Mentha arvensis*)

Japanese Mint oil is distilled from this species.

*Scent:* Strongly mint.

*Components:* It contains such a high percentage of Menthol that the Menthol can be obtained simply by freezing the S-D oil and bottling the crystals. The Menthol content can be up to 90%, and the Menthone content up to 20% with other components. When you can purchase Menthol as a crystal, it makes a fine addition to creams and remedies that are used for coughs, colds, and flus; however, for most uses, Peppermint oil works quite well.

Menthol is considered an antibacterial and a soother for the motor nerves. It is stimulating to the brain but also associated with constriction of the blood vessels. It has been used for sciatica, migraines, headaches, and in blends to discourage all types of vermin. A teeny bit on a sugar cube or in honey can be used for indigestion and vomiting. It is contraindicated for those who are taking homeopathic remedies (it will antidote the remedy), babies, or those with serious respiratory problems where inhaling menthol will cause temporary loss of breathing.

*Properties, Indications, & Uses:* Considered a tonic stimulant, stupefying at elevated doses. Can cause trembling and agitation. Considered an anticephalic. Indicated for: Migraines, headache, and to kill vermin.

*Contraindicated:* Not to be used on babies and children.

***Mentha x citrata*** Common name is **Bergamot Mint**

*Habitat & Growth:* Can be a perennial herb up to 2 feet high with glossy leaves and colorful flowers.

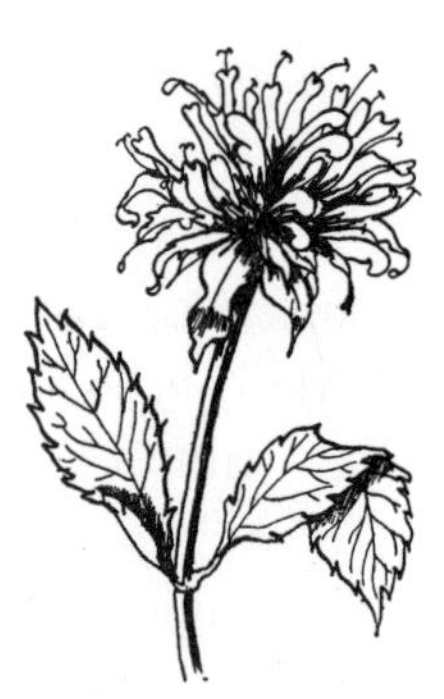

Bergamot Mint

*Scent:* Mint, citrus, and earthy odor.

*Components:* EO S-D from tops but not often found in United States. Mainly Monoterpenes with Linaloöl predominating and Linalyl acetate.

*Properties, Indications, & Uses:* Tonic, for the male sexual system, and antispasmodic.

*Indicated for:* Weakened male sex drive and to ease nervous fatigue.

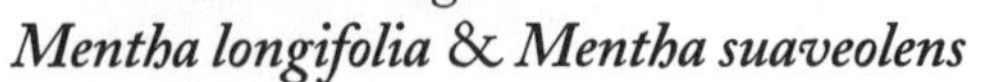

***Mentha longifolia* & *Mentha suaveolens***

This is another Mint oil that is not often found in the United States and will not be discussed.

## Moroccan chamomile (*Chamaemelum mixtum*)

also called **Yellow Chamomile** oil

(See also Camomile)

Ormenis mixta was originally known as Anthemis mixta and is correctly called *Chamaemelum mixtum.*

*Family:* Asteraceae

*Habitat & Growth: C. mixtum* (L.) is described as a somewhat pubescent *annual* 10–60 cm., often much branched with divaricate branches. Found in cultivated fields, roadsides, and maritime sands of the Mediterranean region and southwest Europe and extending northwards to west coast of France. O. mixtum is correctly identified as *Chamaemelum mixtum.* I referred to Arctander's book for fragrance and color of this particular plant. "This plant grows wild and is available in substantial quantities. Moroccan Chamomile Oil, is related to 'German Chamomile' botanically but Ormenis multicaulis, does not at all resemble this plant. It is a good-looking plant, 90–125 cm high with very hairy leaves and tubular yellow flowers. The plant is probably a native of northwest Africa and evolved from a very common Ormenis species which grows all over the Mediterranean countries.[6]

*Scent:* The oil of Ormenis multicaulis *(Chamaemelum mixtum)* has a

[6]Steffan Arctander, *Perfume and Flavor Materials of Natural Origin,* (Elizabeth, N. J.: Steffen Arctander, 1960) p. xx.

fruity and floral herbaceous odor. It is a pale-yellow to brownish-yellow mobile liquid. "The odor of the pale oils, is fresh-herbaceous, slightly camphoraceous, but soon changes into a sweet, cistuslike and rich-balsamic undertone which is very tenacious and pleasant..."[7]

*Components:* Arctander says that the lighter-colored oils are obtained at the beginning of flowering and that towards the end of flowering the oil becomes darker and with a lower yield. Active principles include a-pinene, terpene alcohols, 33% santolina alcohol, yomogi alcohol, camphor ketone and 1,8-cineol oxide terpene. "It presents the highest in alcohol content of these three oils."[8]

*Properties, Indications, & Uses:* Anti-infectious, bactericide against coli-bacteria, parasiticide against worms and amoeba, a general tonic, neurotonic, and aphrodisiac.

*Indicated for:* Problems of the liver and stomach, parasitosis, amoebic cysts, eczema, dermatitis, prostatitis, other sexual problems and disease, nervous depression, and atherosclerosis.

## MQV or True Niaouli (*Melaleuca quinquenervia viridiflora*)

*Family:* Myrtaceae

*Habitat & Growth:* One of the paper bark trees reaching a height of 60 feet. One of two of the paper bark trees that are physiological forms of the same exact species. One form produces MQV EO and the other is called Niaouli EO.

*Scent:* Sweet, woody, herbaceous, and waxy odor.

*Components:* Monoterpenes and Sesquiterpenes.

*Properties, Indications, & Uses:* Provides relief from allergies, bronchitis, laryngitis, and earache. Antiseptic, anti-allergic, and antiviral. It is inhaled to shield against negative energy and protect against a psychic attack.

M.Q. Cineolifera is considered powerfully anti-infectious and antibacterial and is very active on staph germs. It is used for the pulmonary and lymphatic system, an antifungal against candida, and an antiviral. It has hormonelike action on the HPA system as well as the adrenal and ovarian-testicular system.

*Indicated for:* Genital herpes, condyloma, skin lesions, dysplasia,

---

[7]See note 6 page 109, p. xx.

[8]Steffan Arctander, *Perfume and Flavor Materials of Natural Origin,* (Elizabeth, N. J.: Steffen Arctander, 1960) p. xx.

all sorts of vaginal irritations and disease, cancer in those that are not hormone dependant, urethritis, and prostatitis.

M.Q. Nerolidolifera has hormonelike properties and is considered an aphrodisiac. It has powerful action on the HPA.

*Indicated for:* Liver and pancreas difficulties, rheumatoid arthritis, and serious skin disease.

See also Niaouli.

## **Muguet** or **Lily of the Valley** (***Convallaria majalis***)

*Family:* Liliaceae

This beautiful, ornamental flower is up to 1 foot in height with a very sweet fragrance. The rhizome has been used in medicine for the heart, and the flowers are used in scent and snuff. It is considered poisonous and has naturalized to North America. Since the flowers are processed with solvent and are very expensive, it is not found in AT use except where absolutes are used in mind and psyche work.

## **Mugwort** (***Artemisia herba alba*** or ***A. vulgare***)

*Family:* Asteraceae

Common Mugwort is a perennial which grows wild in Europe and Asia. All parts produce EO, but it is not produced commercially. The French use *A. herba alba* and call it Armoise (see below). Often Mugwort is distilled from *A. vulgare* and simply called "Mugwort oil."

*Habitat & Growth:* Wild, weedy looking *Artemisia*, annual or perennial.

*Scent:* An unpleasant blackish, green essential oil with a powerful nauseating herbaceous scent with licorice overtones. The thujone sticks in your nose long after you have inhaled its odor. Very much a thujone/wormwood smell.

*Components:* Up to 55% Sesquiterpenones.

*Properties, Indications, & Uses:* Mucolytic.

*Indicated for:* Certain cancers and chronic bronchitis.

There is another EO called Armoise with 75% Thujone which is much different in qualities than *A. herba alba*. It is used as a mucolytic and parasiticide.

*Indicated for:* Removing warts and internal parasites and in massage oils for aching joints and muscles.

*Contraindications:* Not to be used on babies or pregnant women. Both of these oils are considered neurotoxic and abortive.

## Myrrh (*Commiphora molmol* or *C. myrrha*)

*Family:* Burseraceae

Gum resin obtained from several species of *Commiphora,* includes Abysinnean Myrrh. The taxonomy of the tree which yields commercial gum Myrrh is confused with more than 60 species, all native to Africa and Arabia.

*Habitat & Growth:* Small stunted tree growing wild in various parts of Africa. Incisions made in the bark cause the exudation of oleoresin. Sold as tears and distilled elsewhere.

*Scent:* Hot, smoky, herbaceous, woody, and dry odor.

*Components:* Chemical composition is complicated with several constituents having the characteristic Myrrh odor, probably Sesquiterpenes including Heerabolene.

*Properties, Indications, & Uses:* An ancient balsam used for thousands of years. Forms a very valuable modern ingredient in perfumes. The resinoid is a fixative. Antiviral, hormonelike, moderates the thyroid, anaphrodisiac, and anti-inflammatory.

*Indicated for:* Dysentery, hyperthyroid, and to calm sexual excitement.

*Uses:* A powerful scent used in spiritual work and to excite the upper chakras.

## Myrtle (*Myrtus communis*)

*Family:* Myrtaceae

*Habitat & Growth:* Native to North Africa. Wild evergreen bush which grows profusely in poor soils on sunny hills in Mediterranean. Since antiquity, these aromatic leaves have been highly esteemed and used for perfume and food. There are several types of Myrtle oil: French, Spanish, Corsican, Moroccan, and Italian.

*Scent:* High fruity, herbaceous, and clean odor. A red oil.

*Components:* EO and hydrosol produced from S-D of leaves. Myrtenol, including Nerol.

*Properties, Indications, & Uses:* In the United States we mainly use the hydrosol as an important soothing agent for the eyes, as it can be directly applied. The EO is not often encountered.

Expectorant, skin tonic, and hormone qualities, especially for the ovaries and thyroid.

*Uses:* Tea and EO can be used in bedtime preparations to cure insomnia. Good for oily skin, open pores, hemorrhoids, and external skin irritations. Used in night creams.

### Narcissus (*Narcissus poeticus*)

*Family:* Amaryllidaceae

Several species of Narcissus are grown and extracted for the concrète and absolute which is a very fragrant, waxy mass, that is yellow-green in color and characteristic of the live flowers.

*Habitat & Growth:* Flowers grown from bulbs. About 1 foot in height with heavily scented flowers from white to yellow.

*Scent:* Heavily sweet, floral, green, and salty odor.

*Components:* The components that give the specific scent have not been carefully studied.

*Properties, Indications, & Uses:* Importance in the perfume industry. Blends well with Jasmine. Can be very stupefying. Cut flowers should not be used in the bedroom at night because of this narcotic quality.

### Neroli (C*itrus aurantium ssp. aurantium*)

*Family:* Rutaceae

(See Citrus)

*Scent:* Floral, powdery, and aldehyde odors; a little spicy, maybe green. Yellowish in color.

*Components:* Flowers of this Citrus tree are S-D to produce EO called Neroli. 35% Monoterpenes, 35% alcohol Terpenes, Jasmone, and Nerol which forms its very indicative scent.

*Properties, Indications, & Uses:* Antidepressant and neurotonic.

*Indicated for:* Internal parasites, hemorrhoids, tuberculosis, fatigue, nervous depression, and birthing.

*Uses:* One of the most important of the flower oils as it can be S-D or extracted by solvent. When inhaled, Neroli is antidepressant, a mild sedative, and, when used at night, eases insomnia. In spite of this, it is also joyous and uplifting. It can also be taken internally, *1 drop* in honey for insomnia and diarrhea, or in champagne as an aphrodisiac. Externally it is good for oily or dry skin; it is a facial softener and provides great benefits in overall skin care. It is used in perfumery and as a deodorant.

**Niaouli (*Melaleuca viridiflora*)** See also MQV and Tea Tree
*Family:* Myrtaceae

This is a great substitute for Tea Tree as it is softer and sweeter scented and has the same germicidal and solvent properties. It is used in a variety of skin disorders and infections including skin cancer, chicken pox, cold sores, herpes, acne, and roundworm. It can also be used for strep throat and dental abscesses.

*Scent:* Herbaceous, vegetative like spoiled cabbage, and camphoraceous. Clear to pale yellow oil.

*Properties, Indications & Uses:* This oil is antiinfectious and especially useful for children, as it is more gentle both in scent and action than Tea Tree. It is antiseptic.

*Indications:* Bronchitis as an inhalant, applied to ease burn pain, can be taken in suppository form to protect the immune system from viral infections.

*Uses:* Especially for children and in cases where Tea Tree is not an acceptable scent.

**Nutmeg (*Myristica fragrans* )**
*Family:* Myristicaceae

Both oil of Nutmeg and oil of Mace are included here because they are both derived from the fruit of the same tree. Nutmeg is the dried, ripe seed, and Mace is the dried arrillode (netlike covering) which envelops the shell. Both are important spices and the EO can be used in the flavoring industry.

*Habitat & Growth:* Native to Moluccas, but cultivated elsewhere. An evergreen tree up to 60 feet with dense foliage.

*Scent:* Spicy, warm, and nutty odor. Clear oil.

*Components:* Monoterpene hydrocarbons with Myristicin, among others.

*Properties, Indications, & Uses:* I personally have rarely used either of these EOs because they are very strong and can be irritating, although I have used the ground spice and EO to flavor foods; they are an extremely important part of the food flavor industry.

As a mood lifter for the home: 1 drop of Nutmeg with 20–40 drops of Orange peel oil in a diffuser is wonderful. Nutmeg is considered analgesic and neurotonic.

*Indicated for:* Parasitosis, asthene, extreme tiredness, and aching in the joints (in massage blends). Mace is an analgesic and neurotonic and used in the same manner. It has an additional use of being suitable to facilitate birthing.

*Contraindications:* Use with caution as inhaling this excessively can cause nausea.

**Oakmoss (*Evernia prunastri*)**

*Family:* Usneaceae

*Habitat & Growth:* Oakmoss is not a true flowering plant but a lichen (algae + fungus), which is an epiphyte (a plant which gets nourishment by growing upon another plant) that is extracted for its fragrance. They grow well on trunks of the Oak and Pine, particularly in Europe.

*Scent:* Odors of moss and leather, very smoky. Blackish-brown in color. When the lichen is dried and stored, it develops a peculiar, earthy, mossy odor which is extracted with solvents yielding resinoids, concrètes, and absolutes.

*Components:* Chemical composition of the extracts from both Tree Moss and Oakmoss differ greatly according to the botanical or geographical origin of the lichen, type of solvent used, and method of extraction. *E. prunastri* contains Evernic acid, Usnic acid, and *E. furfuracea* contains other components.

Another lichen which is treated by solvent extraction is Tree Moss or *Evernia furfuracea*. What is called Oakmoss is generally several different varieties of lichen growing together. Occasionally, Usnea is treated by solvent extraction as well› although Usnea is best known for its herbal use in coughs and asthma.

*Properties, Indications, & Uses:* I love Oakmoss, which is really a lichen. Its properties are more emotional and spiritual than physical. It can be used as an addition with respiratory oils as an inhalant to relieve congested sinus; the addition of *Rosemary pyramidalis* would be a good choice.

*Indications:* Indicated as an inhalant for headache or sinus infections.

*Uses:* Primarily used in perfume blends as a powerful and true fixative yielding an earthiness to any blend. It is used ritually for spiritual depth, in incense blends or inhaled by itself to visualize past wounds or hurts, and to increase personal prosperity and cash flow. When inhaling this scent, some people give a "deep gasp of recognition" even though they have never smelled it before.

### **Olibanum** See **Frankincense**

You will generally find Olibanum listed on product lists rather than the higher priced and sometimes different product called Frankincense.

### **Onion (*Allium cepa*)**

*Family:* Liliaceae

Liliaceae family includes Garlic, Onion, Lily, and Lily of the Valley.

*Habitat & Growth:* Native of Asia. Perennial or biennial herb up to 4 feet. Pungently fragrant hollow leaves, flowering stem, and round bulb of many layers used as a food or S-D for a pungent oil.

*Scent:* Pungent, smelly, strong, and sulphurous.

*Components:* Mainly disulfides.

*Properties, Indications, & Uses:* Anti-infectious and reduces catarrh and cholesterol.

*Indicated for:* Infections in the gut or respiratory system and externally in massage blends for rheumatism.

*Uses:* Mainly commercially as an ingredient in flavors for meats, sausages, soups, and many culinary condiments.

### **Opopanax (*Opopanax chironium*)**

*Family:* Burseraceae

Though often confused in the herb world, there is no confusion in the AT world regarding this plant. Common name is oil of Bisabol Myrrh. It is native to the Levant. It is the concrète juice or oleo-gum resin from this plant (which is closely related to Parsnip) that is used; however, what is often found in the marketplace called gum Opopanax is a type of Myrrh and is often confused with true Myrrh.

*Habitat & Growth:* Native to east Africa. A tall, tropical tree con-

Opopanax, also known as Bisabol myrrh and Sweet myrrh, is from the botanical source *Opopanax chironium* Koch (true opopanax). Family: Apiaceae or *Commiphora erythraea* var. *glabrescens* Eng. Family: Burseraceae. Foreign names include Opoponax (French), Opoponax (German), Opoponaco (Spanish), and Opopanax (Italian).

The essential oil is from the oleo-gum resin exudate. Opopanax is an oleo-gum resin that oozes through incisions made on the bark of the tree. The exudate hardens on exposure to air, forming resinous, tear-shaped, more or less regular lumps approximately the size of a nut. These are detached from the bark and used for the manufacture of the essential oil and other derivatives. The trees are native to Somaliland.

*O. chironium* crude resin is offered in the form of regular, tear-shaped lumps of a brilliant red color. They are rather soft, shiny, and easily groundable. The strong, aromatic odor is reminiscent of Costus and Lovage.

The crude oleo-resin has a reddish-brown, or sometimes yellowish-brown, color and sweet, balsamic, slightly spicy odor reminiscent of Myrrh. The material contains 50–80% of a water-soluble gum, 15–40% alcohol-soluble resins, and 5–9% essential oil. The product is also known as bisabol or sweet Myrrh. The adulteration is readily detectable, since Opopanax tears in benzene do not react; Myrrh tears yield a violet color in the presence of bromine vapors.

The oil is obtained by steam distillation of the crude resin in approximately 3.5–10% yields. It is a yellow to greenish-yellow liquid with an intense, warm, and balsamic odor. The oil tends to resinify on exposure to air. Its main constituents include bisabolene ($C_{15}H_{24}$) and a mixture of alcohols. From the oleo-resin, resinoid and resin absolute are obtained. The resinoid, prepared by solvent extraction, is a semisolid mass. To prepare a pourable product, usually a high-boiling, odorless solvent is added prior to evaporation of the extractive solvent. The resin absolute is prepared by direct alcoholic extraction of the crude resin.

The essential oil and derivatives are used extensively in per-fumery because of their good fixative properties. The essential oil is used for flavoring alcoholic beverages (to impart a spicy, warm note) and in some Oriental-type specialties. *—from Herbal Products flyer, 1996*

taining an oleo-gum resin in vessels that occur between the bark and the wood of the trunk.

*Scent:* Warm, biting, sharp, and myrrh-type odor.

*Components:* Resins, gums, and EO, mostly Sesquiterpenes.

*Properties, Indications, & Uses:* Anti-inflammatory and antiparasite.

*Indicated for:* Dysentery, skin ulcers, and parasitical infections in the gut.

*Uses:* Fixative or in incense to retrieve past lives.

## Orange flower

(See Neroli and Citrus)

## Orange peel (*Citrus sinensis* or *C. dulcis*)

*Family:* Rutaceae

See Citrus

*Habitat & Growth:* Native to China. Small, evergreen tree with a deliciously sweet pulp.

*Scent:* Sweet, sugary, citrus odor. Very fresh and high. Pale-yellow to dark yellow-red oil.

*Components:* Extraction by cold expression of S-D of peel. Monoterpenes, mainly Limonene.

*Properties, Indications, & Uses:* Antiseptic and calming.

*Indicated for:* Local disinfection and nervousness.

*Uses:* Externally in skin care. Internally for obesity, water retention, bronchitis, constipation, colds, and flu. Inhaled for nervous tension and stress.

## Oregano (*Oreganum vulgare*)

*Family:* Lamiaceae

(See Marjoram)

There is much confusion in the group of plants that include Thyme, Marjoram, and Oregano (See Marjoram).

*Habitat & Growth:* Common Oregano is native to Europe. Cultivated worldwide. A hearty, bushy herb up to 3 feet. Much used in the world's cuisine.

*Scent:* Herbaceous and somewhat camphoraceous.

*Components:* Any number of constituents including Carvacrol, Thymol, Linaloöl, and Pinene.

*Properties, Indications, & Uses:* We can consider it mainly a painkiller. It is antiviral, fungicidal, parasiticide, stimulant, and tonic for the entire system.

*Uses:* Common Oregano is used in the same way as Marjoram but has a much stronger, more coarse scent. Used in massage blends for aches of the joints.

## Oregano, Spanish (*Thymus capitatus*)

No clear distinction has been made between this and regular Thyme oil.

*Habitat & Growth:* Native to the Middle East. Grows wild in Spain. Perennial, creeping herb.

*Scent:* My experience with this essential oil is from a bottle dating from 1975, my EO library collection. This golden yellow oil smells of Thyme, dried herbaceous bundles of Oregano, and a peculiar fresh shoe-polish odor.

*Components:* Flowering tops are S-D for the strong smelling oil. A variety of constituents including Carvacrol, Thymol, Pinene, etc.

*Properties, Indications, & Uses:* Same as Oregano, above.

*Contraindications:* Can be a powerful skin and mucus membrane irritant and some say should not be used on the skin at all. I purposely put a drop to my nose to see if it was an irritant and sure enough, I got an intense burning sensation on the tissue between the nostrils which then turned bright red. Immediately, I went to the Olive oil and applied it, wiped it off, applied it again and wiped it off. The burning sensation slowly reduced and my nose went back to its normal color. So I have to agree that it is a powerful counterirritant and should only be used highly diluted in carrier oil as a massage for aching joints.

## Ormenis

(See Moroccan Chamomile)

## Orris root

*Family:* Iridaceae

From several species of Iris, including *I. Pallida, I. Florentina,* and *I. germanica.* I have been growing Iris for its Orris root for twenty years. It is the rhizomes of the plant that are used for its powerful fragrance; however, this fragrance takes many years to develop. After the plant has been pulled, cleaned, washed, dried, and stored, the fragrance finally develops. Bugs love Orris root, and in commercial plantings, much of the product is lost to infestation. At home, this can be controlled by storing the roots individually. I have kept them in my desk drawer for three years before I smelled the typical, violet odor.

*Habitat & Growth:* Native to Mediterranean. Grown commercially in Italy. An attractive perennial up to 4 feet. Looks like the typical Iris with delicate, pale blue or white flowers that are deliciously scented. The flowers themselves are not used for their scent, although I believe the home gardener could extract this wonderful aroma by enfleurage.

*Scent:* Warm, toast, powder, and floral odor. Opaque-white to yellow oil.

*Components:* The dried and aged rhizomes are extracted by solvents to yield resinoids, which produce concrètes and butters. These are then S-D for the extraordinarily expensive EO. The fatty Esters are only obtained by very long S-D. Contains 100 or so other components including Myristic acid and Irone.

*Properties, Indications, & Uses:* Mucolytic with particular indications for asthma and chronic bronchitis.

*Uses:* The dried "herb" material from the root is used as a fixative in potpourris. The whole root is used for teething infants. The powdered root is used with Almond meal as a dry shampoo. It is used in face powders as a spot and freckle remover and in shampoo for scalp conditions. This is one of the most important components in making a Violet scent.

*Contraindications:* Can cause serious allergic skin reaction.

## Oud or Aloes wood (*Aquillaria malaccensis* or *agallocha*)

*Family:* Thymelaeaceae

Native to Malasia and named by Jean Baptiste Antoine Pierre Monet de Lamarck (1744–1829). This is the Ahaloth or Aloes wood mentioned in the Bible as "Aloexylum." The decaying heartwood is saturated with a resin, the basis of incense. When distilled it is used in scent and medicine. The fiber is used for rope and textiles. Oud comes in a tiny bottle usually of a brown oil with the name "Agarwood" on the label. "Agarwood" and "Aloewood" are other names for Oud oil, botanically known as *Aquillaria agallocha.*

*Habitat & Growth:* According to Steffen Arctander in his *Perfume and Flavor Materials of Natural Origin,* Agar oil is water distilled from the fungus-infected wood of the *Aquillaria agallocha*, which grows in northeast India. The tree is also found in certain parts of China. Healthy trees have an odorless wood that produces no essential oil. Only older trees are attacked by the fungus and thereafter produce an oleoresin inside the wood. Wood from infected trees is cut and coarsely chopped, then soaked in water prior to distillation. After proper maceration of the wood, this oleoresin will yield an essential oil upon distillation. Being a distillation at atmospheric pressure (100°C), the process of totally exhausting the yield of the wood is a lengthy one. The oil is high boiling and the distillation waters must be cohobated in order to produce a reasonable yield.

*Scent:* The scent is smoky, vegetative, and very ancient.

*Components:* Still being examined.

*Properties, Indications, & Uses:* In Japan, Oud is burned at funerals.

## Palmarosa (*Cymbopogon martinii* var. *motia* syn. *Andropogon martinii)*

*Family:* Poaceae

Closely related to Ginger grass, Lemongrass and Citronella grass.

*Habitat & Growth:* Wild growing herbaceous plant. Native to India; now grown elsewhere. Must be mountain grown to have effective components. Grassy leaves are very fragrant.

*Scent:* Powdery, floral, and herbaceous, smells like fresh cut vegetables Clear oil.

*Components:* Leaves, stalks, and flower heads are S-D yielding up to 1.71% oil. Citronellal, Citral, and mainly Geraniol up to 95%. Commonly adulterated with poor quality Ginger grass.

*Properties, Indications, & Uses:* Antifungal and antiviral with qualities to tonify the heart and has a large spectrum of antibacterial action.

*Indicated for:* Bronchitis, birthing, regeneration of the skin, and regulating oil production of the skin.

*Uses:* Taken internally for virus or bacteria of the gut. Inhaled for cardiac fatigue and virus in the blood. In body care, this is one of the most important EOs. Wonderful for teenagers to regulate oil production of the skin and in the elderly to regenerate and stimulate cellular structure for old, dry, wrinkled skin. Can be used in all blends for skin care. Has a wonderful, sweet, rosy, Geranium odor that makes a wonderful addition to soap blends and cosmetic perfume blends. Moisturizes the skin so is used in creams and lotions. Antifungal, powerful antiviral, useful in AIDs patients to treat Cryptococcus, and protects against influenza. Externally used for acne, wrinkles, scar tissue, and as an analgesic. Inhaled for hypothyroidism. According to Marguerite Maury, it can be used against pathogenic intestinal flora.

### Parsley (*Petroselinum sativum*)

*Family:* Apiaceae

*Habitat & Growth:* A common garden plant native to the Mediterranean and cultivated since antiquity. Was used by the Greeks and Romans in aromatic garlands. Widely cultivated and widely employed in the world's cuisine. Usually biennial and up to 2 feet.

*Scent:* Warm, green, top-of-the-mouth odor that is herbaceous and spicy. Smells like the plant. Pinky-yellow oil.

*Components:* All parts of the plant, especially the seed, contain EO. Parsley seed oil contains a-Pinene, mainly Apiole, etc. Parsley herb oil components seems not to have been identified as yet.

*Uses:* Mainly used in the flavor industry and food production industry. Both herb and oil cause diuresis and so is used for cellulite and taken for toxins, arthritis, flatulence, and indigestion. Used externally to reduce the appearance of broken blood vessels. Whether inhaled or taken seems to aid the labor process. Can be taken for problems of the genito-urinary system. Is a great addition as a carminative in herbal waters used for the digestive system. Forms a particularly interesting green odor in men's fragrances and soaps. Guenther points out that only Parsley herb oil represents the true odor and flavor of the herb we all know so well.

## Patchouli (*Pogostemon cablin*)

*Family:* Lamiaceae

More than 100 years ago when precious fabrics and shawls arrived in Europe from India, they were permeated with an earthy scent, strange at the time, that was characteristic and proof of their origin. About 1844, the first shipment of dried Patchouli leaves arrived in London, and it was then determined that the strange odor of Indian shawls was simply Patchouli. Naturally, astute businessmen in France soon began to perfume their own homespuns with Patchouli and pass them off as the exotic Indian-made fabrics.

*Habitat & Growth:* Native to Asia. A perennial, bushy herb, up to 3 feet with leaves 2–4 inches long and hairy.

*Scent:* Earthy, smoky, spicy and musky scent. Color ranges from dark amber (when S-D in stainless steel) to dark brown.

*Components:* Leaves are dried, cured, and S-D for EO. A roselike odor when aged containing alcohol, Sesquiterpenes, Patchoulene, and Azulene.

*Properties, Indications, & Uses:* Great in skin care as it regulates cellular tissue.

*Indicated for:* All aspects of the skin, especially old skin.

*Uses:* One of the most important and valuable raw materials of the perfume trade. Gives a lasting, alluring quality to any perfume. Very good in all soaps and cosmetics. Acne and seborrheic eczema.

This is one of the EOs that benefits from long storage. When first distilled, the pungency is almost repugnant, and this odor formed the basis of the scent of the unwashed hordes of hippies on Haight Street in the '60s; however, after long storage, even up to twenty years, the fragrance deepens and becomes rich and alluring.

## Pennyroyal

*Family:* Lamiaceae

***Mentha pulegium*** **European Pennyroyal**

***Hedeoma pulegioides*** **American Pennyroyal**

Both plants yield EO closely related in properties and composition.

*Habitat & Growth:* A perennial herb up to 3 feet with the American plant being somewhat smaller. Very aromatic leaves. There are several varieties named according to their location.

*Scent:* Strongly pungent, herbaceous and mint.

*Components:* Tops are S-D for the EO from the fresh or dried herb. Mainly Pulegone up to 90% with Menthone and others. Often used for the manufacture of synthetic Menthol.

*Properties, Indications, & Uses:* Mucolytic, tonic, and stimulant.

*Uses:* Emmenagogue when there is congestion in the pelvis. Often used to bring on the menses, and has some use in menstrual difficulties. It has much value to repel insects on animals and the EO can be used diluted either in alcohol or vinegar as a rub to kill fleas or the herb itself can be used to repel vermin in sleep pillows made of burlap for dogs and cats.

*Contraindications:* Considered an oral toxin and uterine abortive. Many aromatherapists will not use this oil.

## Pepper, Black

(See Black Pepper)

## Pepper, Chilé

(See Chilé Pepper)

## Pepper, California (*Schinus molle*)

*Family:* Anacardiaceae

*Habitat & Growth:* Evergreen up to 20 feet in height native to the America's tropics. The reddish fruit (berries) are aromatic and possess a sweet, spicy odor. Can be used in culinary or substituted for true Pepper.

*Scent:* Pungent, peppery, even a little sweet.

*Components:* EO S-D from berries, smells somewhat like Elemi. α-Pinene, Phellandrene, and Carvacrol.

*Properties, Indications, & Uses:* The French use a species of *Schinus* called *terebenthifolius*. This oil is rarely available in the United States, but it has use as an expectorant when inhaled for bronchitis.

*Uses:* For spicy flavor in various food products.

**Peppermint (*Mentha x piperita*)**

*Family:* Lamiaceae

(See Mint and Corn Mint)

*Habitat & Growth:* Originally a hybrid cultivated between *M. viridas* and *M. aquatica*. It was propagated prior to the seventeenth century and is now cultivated worldwide. This is a perennial herb, up to 3 feet, with underground runners that spread widely. This plant is easy to propagate and should be replanted every year or so as it exhausts the soil. For a good quantity of EO, it should be regularly replanted in a new field from the old cuttings. Peppermint does not develop seed and must be reproduced by cuttings.

*Scent:* When fresh a very minty, hot, but very herbaceous, vegetative back note. The herb and vegetable smell is lost with age. A clear oil.

*Components:* EO is S-D in many areas, including the northwest part of the United States. Up to 48% Menthol, up to 30% Menthone, with other constituents including Cineol and Pulegone. There are many chemotypes and strains of Peppermint, and classification and identification can be difficult without GC (gas chromatograph) MS (mass spectrometer).

*Properties, Indications, & Uses:* Cooling; viricide; tonic; and stimulant, particularly to heart, brain, and pancreas; nerve tonic; somewhat anesthetic; a little decongesting for the prostate; and hormonelike to regulate ovarian hormones.

*Indicated for:* Insufficient liver or pancreas juices, flatulence, belching, headache, migraine, nerve pain such as sciatica, and purulent (itching, stinking) eczema.

*Uses:* Very good to disinfect the air for seriously ill patients with AIDS, senility, or those with high fever. For gas in the stomach, whether human or pets, put one drop in ½ a glass of water and sip slowly. Peppermint diffused will cool any room even if it is very hot. Powerful painkiller in cases of trauma.

*Contraindications:* Not to be used on infants or excessively used. **Do not get near the EYES!!!**

**Petitgrain, Orange leaves (*Citrus aurantium* or *C. sinensis*)**
*Sweet Orange Leaf*
Family: Rutaceae.
(See Citrus and Lemon Petitgrain)
*Habitat & Growth:* Medium height tree with glossy leaves and a sweet-flavored fruit.
*Scent:* When fresh, smells vegetative, floral, dry and a bit leathery. Clear oil.
*Components:* Limonene and Dipentene, δ-Linaloöl, Citral, and many others.
*Properties, Indications, & Uses:* To balance nervous system, antispasmodic, nerves that stimulate untoned muscles, excessive acne, reduce excessive perspiration and greasy hair and skin, and a great toner to all body care products.
*Uses:* Inhaled for nervous exhaustion, fatigue, or stress.

***Pinus spp.***
*Family:* Pinaceae
There is confusion and misinformation amongst users of EOs that family Pinaceae includes **Firs, Spruces, Pines, Cedars**, the **Turpentines**, and other plants that are often considered **Cypress** or **Juniper**. Briefly, family Pinaceae includes only *Picea* (**Spruce**), *Abies* (**Fir**), *Pinus* (**Pine**), and *Cedrus* (**Cedar**). These are *Picea excelsa*, *P. mariana* (**Black Spruce**), *P. abies* (**Norway Spruce**), *Tsuga canadensis*, *T. heterophylla* (the **Hemlocks**), *Pseudotsuga douglasii* (See **Douglas Fir**), *Abies sibirica* (**Siberian Fir**), and *Cedrus atlantica* (**Atlas Cedarwood**, see **Cedar**).
*Scent:* Coniferous, airy, and fruity. Sometimes with a citrus note. Some are woody and vegatative. Clear oils. Mainly the trees that produce the EO that are called **Pine** are *Pinus mugo* (**Dwarf Pine**), *P. palustris* (**Long Leaf Pine**), and *P. sylvestris* (**Scotch Pine**).

***Pinus mugo* (Dwarf Pine needle)**
*Habitat & Growth:* This tree is harvested in the Swiss Alps. It is sturdy and shrublike, is protected by the Swiss government, and is harvested according to particular rules and only at certain elevations. Entire branches including the needles are finely chopped

and thrown into the still for the EO. Combination of bark and needle make up an oil that is both airy and grounding.

*Scent:* The oil has a particularly pungent odor reminiscent of both a bark and needle oil.

*Components:* l-α Pinene, β-Pinene, *l*-Limonene and Sesquiterpenes, Pumiliol.

*Properties, Indications, & Uses:*

*Uses:* In Europe, this plant is used for diseases of the skin and scalp and particularly at healing spas where it is inhaled for ailments of the respiratory organs, including pleurisy and tuberculosis. This is a powerful adjunct in the therapies for all sorts of ear, nose, throat, and lung disorders.

## *Pinus Pinaster* (Maritime Pine)

*Scent:* Conifer with earthy backnote.

*Components:* Contains Mono and Sesquiterpenes. A CT of *Pinus pinaster* contains large quantities of terebenthine which is composed of 62% a-Pinene, and 27% b-Pinene.

*Properties, Indications, & Uses:* This oleo-resin is used as a powerful expectorant, antiseptic, and to oxygenate the air. Good for chronic bronchitis, chronic cystitis, and as an anti-inflammatory for the lungs. Can be used externally in massage blends for rheumatism or aching joints.

*Indicated for:* Infections of the respiratory system. In hot water for steam-inhaling treatments. Mainly used as an aerosol treatment.

*Contraindications:* Possible allergies if used externally.

## *Pinus palustris* (Long Leaf Pine or Turpentine)

See Terebinth

*Habitat & Growth:* Tall, evergreen, up to 150 feet with attractive, reddish-brown, deeply fissured bark and with long, stiff needles that grow in pairs. Used mainly for the distillation of American gum sprits of Turpentine. This is a tall, evergreen tree native to the southeast United States.

*Scent:* Coniferous, woody and pungent.

*Components:* Terpineol, among others.

*Properties, Indications, & Uses:* It has been considered a powerful antiseptic spray and disinfectant, especially in veterinary medicine.

*Uses:* Mainly external use as a massage for arthritis and muscular aches, pains, and stiffness. Natural Turpentine has often been inhaled for asthma and bronchitis. This has been much used in commercial industry to manufacture paint but has now been largely replaced by synthetic Pine oil (synth. Turpentine).

### *Pinus sylvestris* Scotch Pine or Norway Pine

*Habitat & Growth:* Tall, evergreen, up to 150 feet with attractive, reddish-brown, deeply fissured bark with long, stiff needles that grow in pairs. EO is produced mainly in the Baltic states.

*Scent:* A clean coniferous, somewhat turpentine odor.

*Components:* Greatly influenced by geographical origin. Mainly Monoterpenes, Pinene, and some Limonene.

*Properties, Indications, & Uses:* Considered to have hormonelike and cortisonelike qualities.

*Indicated for:* Convalescence. Inhaled for bronchitis, sinusitis, and asthma to tonify the respiratory system.

*Uses:* To balance the hypothalamic/pancreas axis as well as the HPA. Hypertensive and tonic stimulant.

### *Ravensara aromatica* (Ravensare)

*Family:* Lauraceae

*Habitat & Growth:* Native to Madagascar. Evergreen Laurel-type tree also cultivated in France.

*Scent:* Spicy and herbaceous.

*Components:* The aromatic oil is S-D from the leathery clove-scented leaves and sometimes the aromatic fruit as well as the bark. Contains a majority of 1,8- Cineol, a high proportion of Terpene alcohol, $\alpha$ & $\beta$-Pinene, and some $\beta$-Caryophyllene and $\alpha$-Terpineol.

*Properties, Indications, & Uses:* Anti-infectious, strongly antiviral, antibacterial, expectorant, and neuro-tonic.

*Indicated for:* Epstein-Barr/chronic fatigue syndrome, whooping cough, shingles, opthalmic shingles, mononucleosis, hepatitis, and insomnia. Externally as a rub on tired muscles.

*Uses:* This EO, 4 drops diluted with some olive oil, is often taken internally in gastro-resistant capsules. It can be used externally, internally, or by inhalation. A sovereign remedy for sore throat is to put 4 drops on a sugar cube or vitamin C tablet, put under the tongue, and suck slowly.

### Ravensare anise (*Ravensara anisata*)

*Family:* Lauraceae

*Habitat & Growth:* See *Ravensara aromatica* above.

*Scent:* Licorice and anise, spicy, herbaceous, clear, and sweet odor.

*Components:* The volatile oil is obtained by S-D of the bark and contain a variety of Sesquiterpenes, Sesquiterpenols, and Phenols, and Anethol and Chavicol.

*Properties, Indications, & Uses:* Estrogenlike properties, facilitates birth, used as a galactogogue to augment milk secretion, and emmenagogue. When inhaled can be stupefying. Carminative and tonic aperitif. Strong analgesic, cardiac tonic, and lung tonic.

*Indicated for:* Excessive or lack of menstrual cycle. By inhalation for menopause, menarche, and to regulate menstrual cycle. By application for menstrual pain. Regulates skin disorders, especially those due to hormone disorders, acne, and PMS.

*Uses*: Flatulence, gas, and indigestion. Used for angina, palpitations, nervous asthma, and bronchitis.

*Contraindications:* Not to be used on children and pregnant women. Skin irritant when used undiluted. Should be avoided by those with intestinal hemorrhages.

*Other information:* Is now becoming available in the United States. **Possibly Endangered.**

### Rose

*Family:* Rosaceae

Of all the scents used in perfumery, that of the Rose is one of the oldest and best known. For thousands of years poets have been inspired by the delightful aroma of this flower. Historians have given many accounts of the methods by which its alluring scent can be captured. One of the earliest mentions is in the Ayurveda, the series of books on the "good life" written in ancient Sanskrit that may be 7000 years old. In the *Iliad* (chapter 23, V186), Homer describes how Aphrodite anoints the body of Hector with Rose oil (probably an annointment of a Rose-infused unguent). Two thousand years ago, Dioscorides, the Greek, speaks of Rose oil but probably means an unguent of animal fats scented with many thousands of Rose blossoms. (For this method, see *The Aromatherapy Book: Applications & Inhalations* by Jeanne Rose, p. 277.) Two thousand years ago, Nero built a palace with ceilings of fretted ivory and panels that released Rose petals and perfume; one time, so many Rose petals were released that the celebrants suffocated under their weight.

"Subrosa" is a term used for secrets held in private and meaning secrets told under the influence of the Rose. The ancient custom of hanging a Rose over the council table indicated that all spoken underneath was to be held in secret.

Rose pomades were much in use and were prepared by macerating Rose petals in hot fat. First distillation was probably by the Arabs in A.D. 500, although ancient drawings show primitive stills as far back as 10,000 BC. In Persia, such large quantities of Rose water were produced that canals were filled with it, and on hot, sunny days, an oily scum would rise to the surface and be captured in small vials; this was the original Otto of Rose. In the early 1600s, the Turks introduced the Rose industry into Bulgaria where, to this day, the town of Kazanlik is still the home of the best Rose planting and best quality EO of Rose.

*Habitat & Growth:* There are 5000 varieties of Roses, and of these, only a few are called "Old Roses" and are used for the extraction of scent.

***Rosa damascena*** forma ***trigintipetala***, the **Damask Rose** or **Pink Damask Rose.** This Rose is so old that it is unknown in the wild and is probably a hybrid of *Rosa gallica* and *Rosa canina*, the so called Apothecary Rose and Dog Rose. *Rosa damascena* is very fragrant and contains a relatively large amount of EO, which is isolated by S-D or extracted with solvents.

***Rosa alba*** aka ***Rosa damascena alba*** is the **White Rose** or the **White Cottage Rose.** It contains less oil than the Pink Damask and the oil obtained is considered of inferior quality. *Rosa alba* is grown as a hedge around the more fragrant Pink Damask as protection against cold and winds and is used as a boundary marker for individual fields.

***Rosa centifolia*** is the **Pink Cabbage Rose** of history. Grown extensively in Grasse, Southern France, and Morocco, where it is called Rose Demi. *Rosa centifolia* is generally extracted with solvents that yield concrètes and absolutes and is considered to be one of the most important products of the natural flower industry in the Grasse region.

*Collection and Distillation:* Flowers are collected early in the morning and distilled as soon as possible. In the retort, the flowers are just covered with water; no excess water is used. Distillation is very slow but maintained at a lively pace because prolonged action of boiling water is harmful to the EO of Rose. The volume of water in the still should be just enough to carry over the oil into the receiver. A Florentine flask is used to separate the oil from the distillate.

*Scent:* The scent is floral, dry, and woody with a fruity or spicy finish. All absolutes are golden to reddish in color. S-D oils are clear to yellow, and S-D Rose crystallizes when it is cold.

*Components:* Ester number ranges from 7–17. After acetylation, varies from 194–240, meaning the total rose alcohol content is 62–80%. Rose oil is often adulterated with Palmarosa oil to increase the total alcohol content of the Rose oil. In addition, components include *l*-Citronellol, Geraniol, Nerol, Linaloöl, Farnesol, Esters, and up to 300 other constituents.

*General Uses:* Rose oil acts upon the liver, the stomach, and the blood. It is cleaning, regulating, cooling, and antidepressive with powerful effects on female and male sex organs. It increases semen count, is a laxative, and in all aspects of skin care for mature skin, dry skin, and sensitive skin. The ritual aspects of Rose oil are obtained by inhalation methods. It has ancient use in spiritual love and as a source of beauty, joy, happiness, and to unite the spiritual with the physical.

*Properties, Indications, & Uses:* General tonic, powerful neurotonic, aphrodisiac, and tonic astringent.

*Indicated for:* Chronic bronchitis and asthma, sexual weakness in both males and females, frigidity, and impotence.

*Uses:* Used by inhalation, application, and can be taken internally either as Rose water or Rose oil dissolved in honey. For centuries Rose petals have been preserved in honey and used as a sweetmeat as a last course to a fine dining experience.

**Rose Hip Seed oil** *(Rosa eglanteria* aka *Rosa rubiginosa)*
*Family:* Rosaceae

Common name is Rosa Mosqueta, which is not a recognized species.

*Habitat & Growth:* Rose Hips are the fruiting bodies of the Rose that develop after the Rose has been fertilized, petals drop off, the hip (uterus) enlarges, and seeds are formed. The hips are picked when ripe and are very high in vitamin C. The seed is removed and pressed to extract the oil which is often deep red (when some of the fleshy hip is left) or clear.

*Scent:* Fleshy and marine, it often has a strong, almost fishy odor.

*Properties, Indications, & Uses:* It has been found to be a very effective skin treatment. Promotes tissue regeneration. Good for scars, burns, and wrinkles.

*Uses:* Can be used as is or diluted with other vegetable oils and used in blends for skin treatment.

**Rosa Mosqueta** leaves and blossoms have been used in popular medicine for a long time. Until now, the main interest was in its large concentration of vitamin C in its fruit, the Rosehip. Research scientists recently discovered that its seed contains more than unsaturated oily acids, like "Olein" and "Linolen" but also contain vitamin A acid that can be used to treat aged skin, scars, and sunburn.

Rosa Mosqueta is a wild Rose, which is also commonly called Rosa Silvestre, Rosa Montes, and Rosa Coral. It grows in bushy, cold, and rainy areas throughout the world. The primary areas in the United States are Missouri, Wyoming, Nebraska, and the Midwest. In South America it grows in Peru, Chile, and Argentina. It is also found in the Mediterranean.

The highest quality oil is extracted by organic solvents using a combination of 50% Ethanol, 30% water, and 20% cold pressed vinegar. After vaporizing the solvent, brown-yellow crystals remain that show identical structures to vitamin A acid in a concentration of 80%.

Extensive scientific research has shown that vitamin A acid has a positive effect on aged skin, scars, and sunburns. It supports the keratin migration cycle that is responsible for a natural cell regeneration of the skin. After using Rosa Mosqueta for three weeks topically on your skin, an increase of renewed cells in the epidermis is noticed. The cells are also activated to produce more collagen, which after a daily application of fourteen months, makes the skin look smoother, fresher, and more supple. The vitamin A acid also supports the natural process of removing old skin and clearing the hair follicle.

Some experts recommend the application of vitamin A acid for acne; however, it has been most effective in the prevention of early aging of the skin. It is especially recommended for people who are exposed to direct sunlight and/or frequently suffer sunburns. The pain will be soothed and the signs of burning disappear. Experiments are showing that after three weeks of topical application, the wrinkles on the skin surface caused by sunburn disappeared and pigment spots faded. At the end of the fourth month, all wrinkles were gone. The vitamin A acid also helps to renew the skin after surgeries. After three months, scars were softened and the skin became flexible again.

Dr. Bertha Pareja and Dr. Horst Kehl, who published the results of their research about the Rosa Mosqueta in "Cosmetics International" in February 1990, came to the conclusion that the oil that is extracted from the Rosa Mosqueta has all positive effects of vitamin A acid but no negative side effects.

## Rosemary

*Family:* Lamiaceae

The genus *Rosmarinus* includes two species, *R. officinalis* and *R. eriocalix*. Both are used in AT work but mainly *R. officinalis*; its cultivars and chemotypes, is what we will discuss.

*Habitat & Growth:* Native to the Mediterranean. Cultivated worldwide. A shrubby evergreen with short, stiff needles or leaves, and deep, blue flowers, sometimes white. Grows up to 6 feet. In my yard Rosemary is 7 feet high. When I first started my AT work, I read that Rosemary wood had in the past been used in the making of fine lutes. This was unbelievable to me as I had only seen Rosemary with

*Rosemary*

a trunk width of no more than 2 or 3 inches. When I moved to my present home in San Francisco I found a Rosemary bush behind an ancient abandoned Victorian house. The gnarly, twisted trunk was 1 foot in diameter. I assume that this plant was over 100 years old. Unfortunately, the house was soon torn down, the wonderful, ancient Rosemary was smashed into pieces, and an ugly apartment building was built in its place. In any case, now I know that Rosemary can indeed attain a size and width enough to make lutes.

*Scent:* Has a camphoraceous, herbaceous odor. The wild Rosemary has a very fresh odor. Clear to pale yellow oil.

*Components:* Leaves, tops, and flowers are S-D. There are four main CTs of Rosemary, although up to 8 are known to exist. CTs include Rosemary that is high in Camphor, a-Pinene, 1,8-Cineol, Borneol, and Bornyl acetate. Mainly, the following components are found: Pinene, Camphene, Cineol, Camphor, Borneol, and Sesquiterpenes.

Properties, Indications, & Uses: Rosemary is a universal aid in massage and wake-up blends.

*Indicated for:* Internally for arthritis and general weakness. Externally for hair and skin as a tonic. Tea or EO can be used to stimulate liver and gall bladder. Inhaled for loss of memory or mental fatigue. In general, used to stimulate both mind and body.

**Rosemary CT Camphor**. Neuromuscular action that is variable depending on dose. A veinous decongestant and powerful mucolytic. It helps in the production of bile. It is a nonhormonal emmenogogue.

*Indicated for:* Muscular contractions, cramps, myalgia, rheumatism, arthritis rub, hypertension, brain fag, cardiac fatigue, chronic cystitis, chronic gallstones, and all sorts of menstrual irregularities such as amenorrhea or excessive menorrhagia.

**Rosemary CT Cineol**. Expectorant, antibacterial especially on staph or strep germs including *Eschericia coli*, and anticandida.

*Indicated for:* Earaches, sinus-bronchial-pulmonary infections, and all aspects of the ear, nose, and throat.

**Rosemary CT Verbenone**. Powerful mucolypolytic and endocrine equilibriant. Used to regulate the hypothalmic, pituitary, and sexual glands (ovaries and testicles). Verbenone is considered an unknown ketone.

*Scent:* $CO_2$ extract is oily, buttery, rosemary scent excellent for brushing onto garlic bread.

*Indicated for:* Bronchitis, asthmatic bronchitis, viral infections, all types of vaginal infections including the Bartholin glands (two small glands located near the entrance to the vagina), all sorts of sexual problems, nervous fatigue, and depression.

**Rosemary pyramidalis CT Pinene-Cineol.** A conically shaped Rosemary with powerful uses. Expectorant with powerful uses for ear, nose, and throat, particularly as a sinus cleanser.

## Rosewood (*Aniba rosaeodora*)

*Family:* Lauraceae

*Habitat & Growth:* Native to South America. A medium-sized tropical evergreen tree. This tree may be harmfully over-harvested in the rainforests. Continual production of Rosewood oil may be damaging the environment.

*Scent*: Powdery, soft, floral odor.

*Components:* S-D of wood chips. 80–90% Linaloöl, Terpenes, Cineol, Nerol, and Geraniol.

*Properties, Indications, & Uses:* Anti-infectious, antibacterial, antifungal, and tonic stimulant.

*Indicated for:* All respiratory infections from babies to adults and vaginal candida. Inhaled for depression, debility, overwork, and the mucus glands.

*Uses:* The oil has a sedative effect. Used neat on pimples and sores. Can also be used as an antiseptic.

*Other Information:* **Endangered.** Substitute something high in Linaloöl, like Linaloe.

## Sage, Clary

(See Clary Sage)

## Sage (*Salvia officinalis*)

*Family:* Lamiaceae

Common name is Common Sage

*Habitat & Growth:* Native to the Mediterranean. Cultivated worldwide. Evergreen perennial herb up to 3 feet. Several cultivars exist.

*Scent:* Herbaceous, somewhat camphoraceous, and rooty smell. A clear oil.

*Components:* Aromatic leaves are S-D and different types differ in their EO components. 31% Ketones. 15% Cineol. 15% Terpene. 11% Borneols with Esters and Sesquiterpenes. Proportions of these components differ in the various cultivars. True Sage oil has dextrorotation, whereas others rotate left.

*Properties, Indications, & Uses:* Lipolytic, anticellulite, antiviral, and antibacterial for specific bacteria including staphs, streps and pseudomonas. A powerful antifungal including candida. Estrogenlike properties and emmenogogue.

*Indicated for:* Insufficient gall and liver output, viral infections of the nerves, pre-menopause, herpes, and bad circulation.

*Contraindications:* Not to be used on young children and pregnant women. It is tonic and abortive. Considered to cause malformations in babies while in utero. Many prominent AT authorities consider that Sage should never be used at all. I believe it can be used in moderation in massage blends for aching muscles and muscular pain.

## Sage, Spanish (*Salvia lavandulaefolia*)

*Family:* Lamiaceae

Common name is Spanish Sage, but is not to be confused with common Sage grown in Spain.

*Habitat & Growth:* Native to and growing wild in Spain. Evergreen similar to Garden Sage but with narrow leaves.

*Scent:* Herbaceous, clean, camphoraceous, slight thujone back note.

*Components:* Leaves are S-D like Lavender with a scent similar to Spike Lavender. Twenty-five pounds of plant material yields .1 kg. requiring 4 hours to obtain. This is sometimes adulterated with Camphor, Eucalyptus, or Pine oils. Pure Spanish Sage oil contains Cineol, Linaloöl, Linalyl acetate, and Camphor.

*Spanish Sage*

*Properties, Indications, & Uses:* Expectorant and anti-infectious.

*Indicated for:* Chills and various bronchial and sinus infections.

*Uses:* Used to adulterate Spike Lavender oil. Not contraindicated as Common Sage is. Some consider this oil to be a cure-all and uses it to promote longevity. It was used to protect against all types of infection, including plague.

## St. John's Wort (*Hypericum perforatum*)

*Family:* Clusiaceae

*Habitat & Growth:* Native to Europe, naturalized to the Americas as Klamath Weed, where it is controlled by biological means because it is toxic to cattle. Small shrub with yellow flowers that when rubbed produce a red oil.

*Scent:* Herbal, dry, and vegetable. S-D oil is slightly green.

*Components:* Leaves are S-D or the flowers are infused for oil. Monoterpenes, Sesquiterpenes, and many others.

*Properties, Indications, & Uses:* Anti-inflammatory for mucus membranes.

*Indicated for:* Inflamed gut, inflamed kidney tubes, prostatitis, and internal traumas.

*Uses:* To ease traumas of the skin. In massage blends for sore muscles, and neck and back injuries. It is astringent and used in shampoos for dandruff, oily hair, and scalp. In ritual use to balance all the chakras.

*Other uses:* The herb is used as a mood-lifter and to support healthy mental function.

## Sandalwood (*Santalum album*)

*Family:* Santalaceae

Please note that West Indian Sandalwood is in fact *Amyris balsamifera*, which belongs to the family Rutaceae. East Indian Sandalwood is what we will discuss and is not related to West Indian Sandalwood. The common name Sandalwood refers to a variety of trees from different families and there is controversy over the true source; however, the most important "Sandalwood" oil is distilled from roots and heartwood of *Santalum album.*

*Habitat & Growth:* Evergreen tree confined to forests in southern India. Known since ancient times when caravans passing over the deserts of Asia Minor carried Sandalwood to Ancient Greece and Rome to be used for religious purposes. Obtains a height of 60 feet and is actually a hemiparasite plant, as the roots attach themselves to nearby plant roots, obtaining food in this manner and causing the host plant to perish. The tree attains maturity at 60–80 years, at which time it is felled and the heartwood distilled. It is being overharvested at this point and may be seriously endangered.

*Scent:* Honey, syrupy, sweet, woody, floral, and dry. Clear to pale oil.

*Components:* Santenone alcohol about 90%; Sesquiterpenes; and many other components. The Indian government has managed to patent several formulas for synthetic Sandalwood oil (or nature identicals from components of other plants), and it is possible that we in the United States have never smelled pure Sandalwood oil unless we are over the age of thirty. This is a plant that you ought to consider never to use again because of its endangered nature.

*Properties, Indications, & Uses:* Decongestant for the lymph and veinous system. Heart tonic. Can be an aphrodisiac in blends with Jasmine or Rose.

*Indicated for:* Pelvic congestion and cardiac fatigue.

*Uses:* Good use in many perfume blends, massage oil blends, and for skin care of all types; in lotions and baths for its healing and moisturizing properties. Inhaled for nervous tension and as a sedative. It is often used in meditation to open the third eye. It has been used internally to treat cystitis and impotence.

*Ancient Uses:* The treatment of various diseases, particularly venereal disease and especially gonorrhea.

## Sassafras (*Sassafras albidum*)

*Family:* Lauraceae

One of the oldest known American EOs. Native Americans used the herb and taught colonial Americans how to use Sassafras tea as a blood cleanser. Considered a tonic tea in the springtime.

*Habitat & Growth:* Native to eastern part of United States. Deciduous tree, 100 feet in height. All parts are aromatic.

*Scent:* Spicy, herbaceous with a root beer back note.

*Components:* EO S-D from dried bark of root. Leaves are also S-D and produce a Lemon-scented oil, but it is not in commercial production. Up to 90% Safrole and others. Sassafras oil is often sold Safrole-free to be used in flavoring foods. Pure Sassafras oil is also thought to be employed in the manufacture of the drug MDA (methylenedioxymethamphetamine, commonly known as "Ecstasy").

*Uses:* Oil used in dentistry as a disinfectant in root canal surgery. Another oil that is called Sassafras oil comes from a Brazilian tree, *Ocotea cymbarum*. This oil contains up to 93% Safrole and is largely used for the isolation of Safrole and its conversion into Heliotropin. This is not recognized by the USP (United States Pharmacopeia).

*Contraindications:* The oil is highly toxic when ingested and considered a carcinogen and serious irritant.

## Savory

*Family:* Lamiaceae

There are two Savory oils: *(Satureia hortensis)* Summer Savory and *(Satureia montana)* Winter Savory. They are both related in chemical composition and they are both S-D from the flowering herb. Winter and Summer Savory herbs and their oils are valuable in the flavoring of soups, sausages, and canned meats and are an important constituent in spicy sauces.

## Summer Savory (*Satureia hortensis*)

*Habitat & Growth:* An annual herb native to Europe, grows up to 2 feet. Naturalized in North America.

*Scent:* Scent is warm, herbaceous, resin, and softer than red Thyme.

*Components:* Carvacrol, Pinene, Cymene.

*Properties, Indications, & Uses:* Antiparasite, antifungal, and in general a stimulating tonic.

*Uses:* All local infections and weakness of the body.

## Winter Savory (*Satureia montana*)

*Habitat & Growth:* Native to Mediterranean. A bushy perennial up to 2 feet.

*Scent:* Herbaceous and resinous odor.

*Components:* EO mainly produced in Spain. 30% Phenols, 25% alcohols, including Linaloöl, Terpeneol and Borneol.

*Properties, Indications, & Uses:* Antiparasite, major anti-infectious,

general tonic stimulant, pain relieving, circulatory tonic, antibacterial for the bronchial tubes, anticandida, and amoebicide. Both summer and winter savory oils are considered to ease diarrhea, due to the presence of Phenols, especially Carvacrol.
*Indicated for:* Nervous fatigue, hypotension, and malaria or recurrent fevers. Externally for rheumatoid arthritis and inflammation of the lymph nodes.

***Schinus molle***
(See Pepper, California)

## Sea Buckthorn (*Hippophae rhamnoides*)

*Family:* Elaeagnaceae

*Habitat & Growth:* This is a small dioecious tree or shrub of sandy coasts and shingle banks. It yields a yellow dye and has been used as a sauce for meat or fish in Europe.

*Scent:* Fatty, oily, warm, vegetative, and toasty odor. Orange color oil.

*Components:* "$CO_2$ Extract of Sea Buckthorn is generally what is found on the market. This $CO_2$ is from the dried berries of *Hippophae rhamnoides* from Lithuania. The extract is produced by supercritical $CO_2$ extraction under use of natural carbon dioxide with no solvent residues, inorganic salts, or heavy metals (if purchased from a good source). The raw material/extract ratio is 6/1. Extraction output 16.5%. About 30% palmitoleic acid in addition about 10% of unsaponifiable matter containing carotinoids (0.12% corresponding to 1900 IU of provitamin A/gram), alcohols, tocopherols, sterols."*

*Properties, Indications, & Uses:* Palmitoleic acid is one of the main constituents of human skin fat; therefore, Sea Buckthorn has anti-wrinkle and skin softening activity and is wound healing by increasing the granulation. It is useful in cosmetics for skin care preparations and in pharmaceuticals. If purchased from a quality source, the product is 100% natural, contains no carriers, no antioxidants, and no other technical adjuncts, and is not reinforced, blended, formulated, diluted, or stabilized.

---

**from a Prima Fleur flyer, 1997.*

**Seaweed** (from a variety of algae that live in the waters off the coast of France)

*Family:* Various

*Habitat & Growth:* Native to the oceans of the world. Hardy plant that grows in light-filled water near the shore.

*Scent:* Smoky, marine odor, like low tide. Dark green oil.

*Components:* Iodine, water, and mineral nutrients.

*Properties, Indications, & Uses:* This EO is applied to the thyroid area to stimulate the thyroid and assist in weight loss. Apply 1 drop per day to hollow of neck. The Seaweed may be mixed 1:1 with Geranium oil.

*Uses:* It alters temper and has some effect on the mental state so that you have more emotional response.

**Spearmint (*Mentha spicata* or *M. viridis*)**

*Family:* Lamiaceae

See Mint

*Habitat & Growth:* Native to Mediterranean. Common in many parts of the world. Very hardy, perennial herb with bright green fragrant leaves. As with many Mints it quickly exhausts the soil and needs to be replanted regularly via the underground or overground stems.

*Scent:* Sweet, mint, warm odor with fern and herbs.

*Components:* Overground plant is S-D. 3000 lbs. charge requires up to 50 minutes and produces over 10 k. of oil. *l*-Carvone up to 56%; Terpenes; Limonenes; Phellandrenes; and sometimes Linaloöl and Cineol.

*Properties, Indications, & Uses:* Anti-inflammatory, calming, mucolytic, and tonic for the digestive system. When inhaled, has a wonderful ability to create a feeling of joy and happiness. Because of this quality, it makes an excellent addition to blends for stress relief.

*Indicated for:* All sorts of respiratory problems and chronic bronchitis.

*Uses:* Wide application in gums, candies, and dental products but not as often used as Peppermint oil because it does not have as many therapeutic qualities. Inhaled for nervous stress and tension.

## Spikenard (*Nardostachys jatamansi*)

*Family:* Valerianaceae

*Habitat & Growth:* Native to mountainous areas in northern India. Found also in China and Japan. A tender, aromatic herb with a pungent rhizomatous root.

*Scent:* Green, caramel, peas, leather, earthy, and fungal, but sweet smell. Greenish-brown oil.

*Components:* Sesquiterpenes about 93%; especially Jatamanson; up to 20% Valcranone; and other minor constituents.

*Properties, Indications, & Uses:* Very calming, both emotionally and physically, and of special value in serious skin conditions. Powerful antifungal.

*Indicated for:* Psoriasis, insufficient ovarian function, athlete's foot, fungal infections, and emotionally for deep sadness.

*Uses:* All cosmetic products, a powerful oil for gounding, for emotional needs. A "Woman's" oil.

## Spruce (*Picea*)

*Family:* Pinaceae

See also Evergreen

There are a number of different trees that are called Spruce including several that are called Firs.

### *Picea mariana* Black Spruce.

*Habitat & Growth:* Grows in Quebec, Canada.

*Scent:* Conifer, herbaceous, airy, and mossy odor. Clear oil.

*Components:* Include 55% Monoterpenes, including Camphene, $\alpha$-Pinene and $\gamma$-3-Carene, $\gamma$-Bornyl acetate, and Sesquiterpenes. Hormonelike, possibly stimulating the thymus gland. Considered to have corisonelike properties that stimulate the HPA axis.

*Properties, Indications, & Uses:* A general tonic for the system indicated for internal parasites, bronchitis, solar plexus spasms, and excessive thyroid function. Black Spruce has much value in the respiratory system. Possibly this oil is extremely valuable inhaled for asthmatics who take corticosteroids.

*Indicated for:* Bronchitis, parasites, antifungal for candida, prostatitis, solar plexus spasms, asthenic conditions, and excellent for sudden fatigue and exhaustion.

***Picea alba* (White Spruce).** Chemical composition is not the same as Black Spruce. Both White and Black Spruce contain Tricylene. Uses of these oils included in Cedar type blends for technical preparations, room sprays, and deodorants.

***Picea excelsa* Norway Spruce.** Young twigs and leaves are S-D. Produced in the Tyrol valley. Very fragrant odor. Not often used. Chemical composition is mainly Pinene, Phellandrene, and Dipentene. It is used in all sorts of Pine-scented compositions, bath salts, room sprays, etc.

**Hemlock-Spruce.** Includes *Tsuga canadensis* (Eastern Hemlock); *Tsuga heterophylla* (Western Hemlock, Grey Fir, Alaskan Pine); *Picea mariana* (Black Spruce); and *Picea glauca* (White Spruce). They are widely known in North America. These trees are tall evergreens with horizontal branches and finely toothed leaves. The young branches and leaves are S-D. Production is normally in the northeastern part of United States. Inhaled for the respiratory system.

## Star Anise (*Illicium verum*)

*Family:* Magnoliaceae

Should not be confused with oil of Anise.

*Habitat & Growth:* Native to southeast Asia. An evergreen tree, 30 feet high with a star-shaped fruit containing many seed-bearing follicles. Very fragrant, but not as finely scented as Anise seed, which is an annual herb.

*Scent:* A clear oil with a strongly spicy, licorice-like odor.

*Components:* Seeds are S-D. Similar composition to Anise seed and Fennel seed oil, including Anethole and about 100 other components.

*Properties, Indications, & Uses:* Antispasmodic and estrogenlike qualities.

*Indicated for:* Colitis spasms and premenopause.

*Uses:* Flatulence, burping, gut spasms, and coughs. Inhaled for menopause possibly to balance hormonal output and to cool hot flashes. Used as a basis to isolate Anethole. Used to flavor cough syrups, cough drops, liqueurs, and aperitifs, although Anise seed oil is more often used. Also used to scent soaps and other body care products. Guenther mentions that animals like the flavor of Anise; therefore, this oil is often used in animal feeds.

**Styrax (*Liquidamber styraciflua*) American Styrax**

*Family:* Hamamelidaceae

*Habitat & Growth:* Native American tree. Reaches a height of over 100 feet. Balsam was used by Native Americans who introduced it to Spain via Cortes. Was used as a perfume and vulnerary. The balsam originates as a pathological product in secretion reservoirs of old trees. Not all *Liquidamber* trees produce this balsam.

*Scent:* Sharp, hot, biting, honey, and aldehyde odor. Smells like benzoin with a leathery note.

*Components:* Balsam is S-D to produce EO. Styrene; Cinnamic acid; Cinnamyl alcohol; Vanillin.

*Properties, Indications, & Uses:* Cicatrix, which helps to close wounds, and pulmonary antiseptic.

*Indicated for:* Skin conditions such as acne, eczema, psoriasis, chilblain, and frostbite.

*Uses:* Medicinal preparations such as tincture of Benzoin. Used to isolate Cinnamyl alcohol and to scent soaps. Powerful odor fixative in perfumes.

**Tagetes (*Tagetes spp.*)** Common name is **Marigold**

*Family:* Asteraceae

*Tagetes glandulifera* is called Mexican Marigold. Scents have been used as a deterrent to house flies as a repellant.

*Habitat & Growth:* Strongly scented annual herb up to 2 feet in height. Bright orange flowers with a strong scent. Very similar to Calendula.

*Scent:* Mint, oily, and fruity odor. A clear, orange-colored oil. Has a powerful, green, intense, sweetish odor. Absolute is dark yellow or dark orange and sometimes turns somewhat green.

*Components:* EO S-D from entire flowering herb or an absolute and concrète by solvent extraction. b-Ocimene; Ketones which includes up to 40% Tagetone; and many others.

*Properties, Indications, & Uses:* Antifungal and antiparasite. Kills round worms in the gut.

*Indicated for:* Respiratory infections and parasites in the gut.

*Contraindications:* Not to be used on pregnant women and children. Considered a neurotoxic and abortive. Arctander states that Tagetone may be harmful to humans. Excessive skin use is discouraged, as it can cause serious photosensitivity.

***Tanacetum annuum***
(See Blue Tansy)

**Tangerine** See Citrus and Mandarin.

**Tarragon (*Artemisia dracunculus*)**
*Family:* Asteraceae
Common name is Estragon
*Habitat & Growth:* Eurasian perennial growing to a height of about 2 feet. Cultivated in Southern France.
*Scent:* Licoricelike, basil, vegetable, and warm, herbal odor. A very eponymous scent. A clear to pale-green oil.
*Components:* Leaves S-D. Methyl Chavicol and probably Ocimene; up to 70% Estragole.
*Properties, Indications, & Uses:* Neuromuscular antispasmodic, antiviral, antiallergenic, and can be an abortive as it stimulates menstrual flow.
*Indicated for:* Spasms of the gut, belching, premenstrual syndrome, abnormal tendency to convulsions, *anorexia*, to balance nervous system, digestive problems caused by emotional distress, and chronic fatigue.
*Uses:* Blends well with earthy odors such as Labdanum, Oakmoss, and Galbanum. Wide use as a flavoring ingredient in fine foods.

**Tea Tree (*Melaleuca alternifolia*)**
*Family:* Myrtaceae
(See MQV and Niaouli)
*Habitat & Growth:* Hundreds of species of *Melaleuca* occur in Australia. A small tree or shrub with narrow leaves and papery bark.
Scent: Clear, shoe polish (aldehyde), herbaceous, and leathery odor with a greenness to it. Smells fungal like spent feet.

*Components:* EO S-D from leaves. Terpinene-4-ol up to 40%; and many other components.

*Properties, Indications, & Uses:* This oil possesses a high germicidal value, has a pleasant if somewhat medicinal odor, is nonirritating and noncorrosive, and has extensive applications in medicine and veterinary medicine. Has the property to penetrate pus and by mixing with it, the pus liquifies which causes it to slough off, leaving a healthy surface. This oil has been extensively written about in *The Aromatherapy Book: Applications & Inhalations* by Jeanne Rose. Many authors mention many properties and indications: immune stimulant, protective against radiation, a major anti-infectious and anti-bacterial agent with a spectrum of action, anticandida, antiviral, and antiparasite, including roundworms.

*Indicated for:* Bacteria and parasites in the digestive system; candida; viral infections; ear, nose, and throat infections; all infections of the genital or reproductive tract for both men and women; local anesthetic after shocks, kicks, or hits; and prevents radiation burns or scalds.

*Uses:* This oil has such a large spectrum of action. It can be used internally, externally, by inhalation, and by application. Can be used on animals, though always use this oil very freshly distilled, as there is some evidence that old Tea Tree oil can cause temporary paralysis in animals. Special care should be taken with cats.

## Terebinth (*Pinus palustris* and *Pinus pinaster*)

*Family:* Pinaceae

(See Pine)

Common name is Essence of Turpentine

Generally, American species that produce Turpentine are *Pinus palustris*, Long Leaf Pine. The French use *Pinus pinaster* to produce Terebinth or Turpentine for therapeutic use. Terebinth SD from resin of the bark.

*Habitat & Growth:* Tall, attractive evergreen with long needles. Various species are native to all parts of the world.

*Scent:* Smoky, coniferous scent.

*Components:* S-D from leaves. [Pine oil = Contains up to 60% α-Terpineol; up to 25% other Terpineols; Borneol; Terpene hydrocarbons, etc.] Terebinthene = 63% α-Pinene; 27% β-Pinene.

*Properties, Indications, & Uses:* Not often used therapeutically by people of the United States. French use it as antiseptic, expectorant, to oxygenate the blood after ozone therapy, and as a stimulant. Pine oil and Turpentine are powerful germicides.

*Indicated for:* Respiratory catarrh and infections. Inhaled for fainting spells.

*Uses:* To scent rooms and clean the air, to inhale as a respiratory disinfectant.

## Thuja (*Thuja occidentalis*) See **Evergreen** and **Cedar**.

*Family:* Cupressaceae

Common names are Cedar leaf , White Cedar leaf, and White Cedarwood oil.

*Habitat & Growth:* Thuja oil is produced only from the leaves of *Thuja occidentalis.* It should not be confused with Cedar leaf oil which is from a Juniper or Cedarwood oil from Thuja. Thuja is a pyramid-shaped conifer up to 60 ft. with scalelike leaves.

*Scent:* Woody, fruity odor.

*Components:* S-D from needles. δ-α-Pinene; δ-α-Thujone, the chief constituent. Fenchone; Borneol, and acids.

*Uses:* Used in Pine and Cedar blends to scent the room. The oil from the boughs is used as a mucolytic; for warts, herpes, and tumors; and to close wounds.

*Old use:* As an official medicinal preparation as a counterirritant.

*Contraindicated:* Use externally only. It is considered a neurotoxic and abortive when taken internally.

It is important that one not confuse the oil from White Cedarwood *(Thuja occidentalis)* with Red Cedarwood *(Juniperus virginiana)* or True Cedar of the genus *Cedrus.* or with Western Cedar, *Thuja plicata..*

## *Thuja plicata* (Western Red Cedar)

*Family:* Cupressaceae

This contains a highly volatile and poisonous Ketone which is very fragrant. Should not be used at all.

## Thyme

*Family:* Lamiaceae

Generally, Thymes are meant to include *Thymus vulgaris* but other species are also included with the Thyme oils. Thymes produce very specific chemotype oils, each with a preponderance of the chemotype after which it is named. The chemotypes include:

*T.* CV. ***Geraniol*** which has a large spectrum of action. It is an antifungal, powerful antiviral, uterine tonic, neurotonic, and heart tonic.

*Indicated for:* All problems of the ear, nose, throat, and lungs, in particular for bronchitis and otitis. The Geraniol chemotype, as with any EO containing large amounts of Geraniol, is useful in urethritis, cystitis, vaginitis, cervicitis, and any inflammation of the female reproductive system. It also is used in birthing. Externally, it can be used for skin disease such as that caused by staph infections or staph acne and eczema. Also useful for viruses in the blood.

*T.* CV. ***Linaloöl*** with up to 80% Linaloöl, this EO is useful as a fungi-cide against candida, either in the stomach or in the gut. It is also used for parasites in the gut and nervous fatigue.

*Scent:* Warm, herbaceous, floral, and powdery odor.

*T.* CV. ***Paracymene*** the composition is mainly Paracymene with some Thymol. It is a pain reliever when used on the skin and is excellent in massage blends for rheumatism and arthritis.

*T.* CV. ***Thujanol*** this chemotype is a powerful antibacterial, particularly against chlamydia, and a strong viricide. Used for problems of the stomach including gas, digestive problems; insufficient liver enzymes; and diabetes. Used for inflammation of the glans of the penis and all external problems of the female and male reproductive system including condyloma, venereal warts, prostatitis, and inflamed skin.

*Indicated for:* All problems of the ear, nose, throat, bronchial tubes, stomach, and external genitalia.

*T.* CV. ***Thymol*** this is a major anti-infectious agent with a large spectrum of action indicated for all local infections; however, *use with extreme caution as it can be caustic to the skin.*

The Thyme family includes a number of species and cultivars with a variety of chemotypes:

*Caution*

Can cause skin burning. There can be a great deal of confusion with the **Thyme** oils due to the numbers of chemotypes. Mainly, Thymol and Carvacrol are warming and active. Thujenol is antiviral and penetrating. Citral and Linaloöl are sweet-scented and nonirritating. The toxic Phenols, Carvacrol and Thymol, are irritating to the mucus membranes and can irritate the skin. They should be used, if used at all, in moderation and heavily diluted with carrier substances.

**Spanish Thyme**. Thymol type; up to 60% Phenol, mainly Thymol. Under this classification you will find Spanish Thyme *(Thymus vulgarus)* and *(Thymus zygis)* both growing wild in Spain. They contain large quantities of Thymol.
**Origanum**. Carvacrol type; up to 74% Phenol, Carvacrol.
**Lemon Thyme**. Citral type.
**White Thyme oil** *(Thymus vulgaris)* can contain large amounts of Phenol and begins to turn red when aged. This is also called Red Thyme.
**Moroccan Thyme oil** is also occasionally called Red Thyme oil.
**Lemon Thyme oil** *(Thymus hiemalis)* contains up to 34% Citral. The new Ketone $C_{10}H_{16}0$ which is called Verbenone. See Rosemary verbenone.
***Thymus hirtus*** is related to ***Thymus hiemalis*** and can contain up to 25% Limonene; Citral; free alcohols; and Fenchone.
**Wild Thyme oil** ***(Thymus serpyllum)*** also called Essence of Serpolet grows wild in southern Europe, contains para-Cymene and other components. Properties are antiseptic, stomachic, neurotonic, and general tonic stimulant.
*Indicated for:* Infections of the gut, general fatigue or nervous fatigue, asthma, emphysema, tuberculosis, upper urinary tract infections, cystitis, and certain skin problems such as impetigo or infected skin disease.
***Thymus mastichina*** Cineol type (Wild Marjoram). With a large quantity of Cineol and a large variety of other chemical components, this particular Thyme is used primarily to decongest the lungs and bronchi. It is an expectorant that stimulates the mucus glands.

*Indicated for:* Bronchial catarrh.

***Thymus satureioides*** type Borneol-carvacrol. This is a powerful immune system modulator and to help *bulimia.* General tonic for the entire system and an aphrodisiac. Used for chronic infections, tuberculosis, general fatigue, sexual weakness, and for persons with weak constitutions.

*Scent:* A clear, hormonal, meaty, herbaceous, and pungent odor.

*Uses:* "Oil of thyme, a powerful germicide, finds wide application as a disinfectant and antiseptic of rather pleasant odor. It is used as such in many Pharmaceuticals and oral preparations—gargles and mouth washes, for example. The oil is said to cause mental excitement; it serves as a diffusible stimulant in collapse. Oil of thyme is used also for the scenting of soaps. On an increasing scale, oil of Thyme serves for the flavoring of all kinds of food products, meats, sausages, sauces, and canned foods, in which it replaces the botanical as a condiment."[9]

## Tuberose (*Polyanthes tuberosa*)

*Family:* Amaryllidaceae

*Habitat & Growth:* Native to Central America and Mexico. Cultivated in Grasse and Morocco. Mentioned in the ancient Aztec Codex. A tall, slender, perennial up to 3 feet with long leaves, tuberous root, and very fragrant, white flowers. In cultivation the bulb has to be replanted every several years. In my experience here in San Francisco, bulbs need to be planted in a sheltered greenhouse with 12 hours a day of sunlight and circulating air from beneath, but no wind, and replanted every other year. After the flowers are harvested, the leaves are allowed to die down, and the pots are put in a dark place until the Spring Equinox. Commercially in the field, the bulbs are dug up in November, stored over the winter in airy, dry places, and replanted in April. There is a single and double variety of Tuberose, the single being the most fragrant.

*Scent:* Strongly floral, earthy, fatty, and tropical scent. A dark, red-amber absolute.

*Components:* Extraction is done by enfleurage or by solvent extrac-

[9]Ernest Guenther, *The Essential Oils,* Vol. III (Malabar, Fla: Kreiger Publishing, 1976) p. 757.

tion and, as with many thick-leafed flowers, the natural scent continues to develop for up to 24 hours after they have been harvested. In modern times, extraction is done strictly by solvent extraction to produce a concrète and absolute of Tuberose. It is one of the most valuable and expensive fragrances known.

Methyl Benzoate; Methyl Salicylate; Methyl Anthranilate; alcohols such as Geraniol and Nerol. Also, an unidentified Ketone $C_{13}H_{20}0$ called Tuberone

*Enfleurage:* Freshly picked flowers, closed, are placed on the chassis, kept 48 hours, and replaced by new flowers. One kg. of corps is treated with 3 kg. of flowers. Approximately 150 kg. of flowers yield 1 kg. of absolute of enfleurage. The residual flowers, when removed from the chassis, still contain some natural and developing flower oil. These are submitted to extraction with petroleum ether and gives the so-called absolute of chassis.

*Properties, Indications, & Uses:* In general it is narcotic and aphrodisiacal.

*Indicated for:* Impotence and frigidity and to induce relaxation.

*Uses:* Mainly by inhalation. Wonderful in expensive perfumes. Can be used to flavor sweets, and 1 drop to a bottle of champagne creates a powerful aphrodisiac.

Since a S-D is not available, it is most often grown at home and extracted by enfleurage or infused in oil. Probably one of the most expensive natural flower oils.

## Turmeric (*Curcuma longa*)

*Family:* Zingiberaceae

*Habitat & Growth:* Native to Southeast Asia. A perennial, tropical herb which grows up to 3 feet. It has a thick, rhizomatous root that is deep orange. After the root is harvested, it is cured in deep pits where the chemical composition develops. It is cleaned, boiled, sun dried, and steam distilled for EO.

*Scent:* Strongly herbaceous, fern, aldehyde, and strongly expansive scent. A pale, clear oil.

*Components:* Root is S-D for EO. 58% Turmerone, about 6% Sesquiterpene alcohols, 25% Zingerbirene, and others.

*Properties, Indications, & Uses:* Pain relieving and aphrodisiacal.

*Indicated for:* Externally for massage and rheumatism. Internally for parasites.

*Uses:* Tea of the root or encapsulated ground root has been found to be of great value as an anti-inflammatory for use in arthritis and rheumatism. It has some of the same uses as the adrenal gland function.
*Contraindications:* Not to be used on babies, children, and pregnant women.

There are other *Curcuma* oils available. These include *Curcuma aromatica,* which is not produced on a commercial scale; *Curcuma domestica,* which is native to Indonesia and used in native medicines for liver and gall bladder disease and also not produced commercially; and *Curcuma zedoaria* (Zedoary oil), which is used in France as a carminative and to stimulate the digestive system and contains Sesquiterpene alcohols with Camphene, Cineol, and Camphor.

## Turpentine

See **Terebinth**

## Underarm odor

The scent can be used to regulate and harmonize the menstrual cycle.

This is one of those plants that it pays the home consumer to purchase whole, as Vanilla is so heavily adulterated and synthesized. It is quite easy to make your own tincture of Vanilla for home use in massage and inhalation: simply take a handful of the long, 6-inch Vanilla beans, split them lengthwise, chop them, and immerse them in an equal amount of full-strength 195% ethyl alcohol or potable rum, just enough to cover the beans and infuse until the fluid takes on the flavor and color of Vanilla. This can then be used in blends. The blends need to be made with the Vanilla and allowed to age, at which time the other essential oils are decanted off, leaving the Vanilla seeds behind, and the alcohol will carry the fragrance of Vanilla with it.

## Vanilla (*Vanilla planifolia* or *V. fragrans*)

*Family:* Orchidaceae

This is the only plant of the Orchid family used in AT work.
*Habitat & Growth:* Native to Central America. Cultivated in many

places. A perennial, herbaceous vine up to 75 feet that is trained to grow in rows. The green fruit which looks like a green bean is picked after it spends some time on the vine and is then cured. This is another one of the plants that has no odor; the odor develops upon drying and curing (See Orris and Patchouli). These immature pods are then picked, put on trays, and left to ferment. When they turn brown and become extremely fragrant, the fermentation process allows the Vanillin to develop, and the best quality beans accumulate white Vanillin crystals on the bean.

*Scent:* Floral, rich, sweet, soft, warm, honey, waxy, hay, and balsamic scent. Oil can be creamy yellow to dark blackish-brown.

*Components:* Vanillin and many other constituents.

*Uses:* Vanilla has powerful uses as an aphrodisiac, in perfume blends, and to flavor and fragrance anything. It has been used particularly to flavor tobacco, ice cream, and chocolate.

**Verbena** ***Aloysia triphylla*** is the true **Lemon Verbena or** ***Lippia citriodora***

*Family:* Verbenaceae

There is much confusion in the literature as to what constitutes Verbena oil. Often a species of Thyme, particularly Lemon Thyme from *Thymus hiemalis* is used. I have found in my practice that often *Litsea cubeba* is also sold as Lemon Verbena.

*Habitat & Growth:* A native of South America, particularly Chile. Found extensively in Europe. Grows well in California as far north as San Francisco. A perennial shrub up to 30 feet. Can develop a very thick, gnarled trunk. Produces a myriad of flowers, small, white in whorled, axillary spikes or terminal panicles (tiny, white flowers) with an intense sweet scent. But it is the leaves and the immature flowers which are S-D in May. When the leaves are S-D with the flowers, the oil takes on a sweet scent in addition to the Citral scent. Can also be distilled in June and July. The distillate has little EO, but much powerful, sweet hydrosol that has all the therapeutic activity of both the herb and the EO.

*Scent:* Green, vegetative, herbaceous, warm, floral scent with some lemon and citrus notes.

*Components:* Distillation yields only up to 0.2% oil. Mainly 35% Citral with other components. The yield is mainly hydrosol.

*Properties, Indications, & Uses:* Powerful anti-inflammatory; fever reducer; powerful sedative when taken either as herb tea, hydrosol, or EO inhaled; and has hormonelike action on the thyroid and pancreas.

*Indicated for:* Stress, insomnia, depression, nervous fatigue, and herb tea for Crohn's syndrome, an inflammatory disease involving the lower portion of the small intestine.

*Uses:* To prevent asthmatic crises. EO is very expensive and not much is available. What is found on the market is composed mostly of Citral, *Litsea,* or mixtures of lemony-scented oils. The hydrosol is especially valuable as a skin toner to reduce inflammation and for all the situations indicated above.

## Vetivert (*Vetiveria zizanioides*)

*Family:* Poaceae

*Habitat & Growth:* Native to India. Cultivated in other tropical places. A perennial grass. Very fragrant, with many underground rootlets. It is these rootlets that are S-D after they have been picked, washed, chopped, dried, and soaked. It has been much grown in the southern part of the United States. EO produced in many countries.

*Scent:* Sweet, woody, caramel and smoky smell. Golden-brown oil.

*Components:* S-D of roots for EO. Ketonic Sesquiterpenes called Vetivone; Vetivenols and other fractions named Vetivert or Vetivone or Vetivene.

*Properties, Indications, & Uses:* Good for circulation.

*Indicated for:* Depression and the immune system.

*Uses:* Bath oils for its relaxing effect, moth repellants, and perfumery. A great substitute for the endangered Sandalwood. In skin care, it is valuable for oily skin and acne.

## Violet flower and leaf (*Viola odorata*)

*Family:* Violaceae

In the past the flower scent was extracted by maceration in hot fat, but now only the leaves are used.

*Habitat & Growth:* Native to Europe and Asia. Cultivated worldwide. A small tender perennial with heart-shaped leaves and very

For perfume work, mainly the Parma Violet and Victoria Violet are used. There is no S-D of Violet flowers. The leaves are extracted by a solvent for a concrète and absolute which is a deep green color with a very earthy, green scent.

The scent of Violet flowers is very evanescent, and as soon as you are able to detect the fragrance, it disappears. What happens is the scent paralyzes the nasal cilia so that they are unable to detect scent. One has to walk away from the Violet and come back to it to be able to experience once again this very particular fragrance.

fragrant flowers. It has an underground rhizome that can spread wildly and take over a yard.

*Scent:* Violet leaf has a stemmy, herbal, sweet, green scent with some woody, floral notes.

*Scent:* Violet leaf has a stemmy, herbal, sweet, green scent with some woody, floral notes.

*Components:* Leaf oil contains Parmone; Eugenol and Violet leaf extracts.

*Uses:* The flower and leaf tea has had much use in herbalism to cure afflictions of the throat. Home use of flower and leaf tea is as a wash for acne, eczema, to refine pores, taken as a tea for bronchitis and throat infections. Inhaled, the flower is used for insomnia and energy slumps. As an adjunct in high-quality perfumes. Both herb tea and extract are used on the throat to treat cancers.

### Wintergreen (*Gaultheria procumbens*)

*Family:* Ericaceae

See Birch

*Habitat & Growth:* Native to North America. Small evergreen creeping herb up to 1 foot in height, with leathery leaves. Plant is collected by hand. Oil of Wintergreen has been synthesized for such a long time that most have never smelled the true oil. It is powerfully sweet and Birch-like but with chewing gum overtones. With a developed sense of smell, one can detect the difference between Wintergreen syn. and Wintergreen EO.

*Scent:* The scent is almost identical to Birch, woody and wintergreen.

*Components:* Leaves S-D for EO. Up to 90% Methyl salicylate.

*Properties, Indications, & Uses:* Antispasmodic and anti-inflammatory.
*Indicated for:* Massage oil blends for rheumatism, arthritis, and any muscular ache or pain.
*Use:* Wintergreen oil synthetic is used to flavor gums, candies, soft drinks, and medicinal preparations, especially those for the teeth and muscles.
*Contraindications:* Can be considered toxic, irritating, and sensitizing as well as a hazard to the environment and a pollutant to marine life.

## Witch Hazel (*Hamamelis virginiana*)

*Family:* Hamamelidaceae
*Habitat & Growth:* Native to United States. Large perennial shrub. Yellow, fragrant flowers, producing catkins. This shrub is deciduous. What is interesting about this plant is that on steam distillation, an EO is not produced; however, the distillate, or hydrosol, is an aromatic water very popularly known as Witch Hazel hydrosol, or extract if it is mixed with 5% (95%) alcohol. This is used as an aftershave and in other body care preparations. Not much is known about the molecules that provide fragrance to Witch Hazel.
*Scent:* Light, woody, herbaceous, aldehydic odor.
*Components:* Leaves S-D. Has been observed that molecules and Esters are produced as well as phenols with an odor somewhat like Eugenol as well as Sesquiterpenes and waxes.
*Uses:* Has wide use as a simple toilet water. The tea of leaves is used in hair preparations and body care products as an astringent.

## Wisteria (*Wisteria sinensis*)

*Family:* Fabaceae
These very fragrant flowers can be infused in oil at home. The flowers are very fragrant with a honeylike scent. Flowers have been extracted with solvent to produce a concrète, but nothing else is known about the fragrance or the composition.

## Wormwood (*Artemisia absinthium*)

*Family:* Asteraceae
The principal constituent is Thujone and because of this toxin,

should not be used in therapy internally or externally. The absinthium has a bad reputation in the late 1800s as the principal ingredient of Absinthe, an alcoholic beverage that caused addiction and mental derangement but also was used by the great painters of that time. Since this oil contains azulenes, is very dark in color, and the plant itself looks very much like *Artemisia arborescens,* it sometimes contaminates distillations of *Artemisia arborescens.* Be wary!

## Yarrow (*Achillea millefolium*)

*Family:* Asteraceae

Common name is Milfoil

*Habitat & Growth:* Native to Europe and Asia. Perennial herb with a single stem up to 3 feet high with lacy leaves and white flowers packed on a flower head.

*Scent:* Dry, herbaceous, but not sweet, and with some thujone odor. Pale yellow to brilliant blue oil.

*Components:* Ketones; Camphor; Lactones; Sabinene; Pinenes as well as up to 51% Azulene which gives it a clear, pale blue color.

*Properties, Indications, & Uses:* Anti-inflammatory. Flower tea is an emmenagogue.

*Indicated for:* Problems of prostate or menstrual problems and neuralgia.

*Uses:* Because of the content of Azulene, Yarrow oil is used in skin care for acne, eczema, and inflammation to minimize varicose veins and reduce scars. Herb tea has much value in cosmetic care. For uses, see *The Herbal Body Book* by Jeanne Rose.

## Ylang-Ylang (*Cananga odorata*)

*Family:* Anonaceae

(See Cananga)

*Habitat & Growth:* Native to Molucca and the Philippines. Tall, tropical tree, up to 60 feet with large, up to 6-inch, very fragrant flowers. Grows in Florida on the University of Miami campus, as well as in the Fairchild Tropical Gardens. This tree occurs in two distinct forms. On S-D the flowers of *Cananga odorata* forma *macrophylla* produce the oil called Cananga oil and *Cananga odorata* forma *genuina* produce the oil called Ylang-Ylang. For an extensive history of this wonderful flower, read Guenther *The Essential Oils,* vol. V, p. 277.

*Scent:* Extra has a fatty, tropical, fruity, floral odor and is a yellow to rich yellow-gold oil. When the flowers are put in a vase at home, the fragrance can last up to a month, even until the flowers themselves are totally dried and shriveled.

*Components:* There are several grades or qualities of EO obtained in the distillation process. The first fractions of oil that are carried over by the steam contain the most aromatic and valuable constituents (Esters and Ethers) of the oil of Ylang-Ylang flowers. The later fractions bring over Sesquiterpenes and other components; therefore, there is a gradual lowering of the fragrant quality of the oil and so the oil consists of "extra," "first," "second," and "third" qualities. For aromatherapy use, you must purchase either "extra," "first," or "second." In order to obtain extra quality, these rules must be followed in the distillation:

1. Only fully mature, yellow flowers are harvested early in the morning.
2. Flowers must not be damaged in picking.
3. Flowers must be immediately taken to distillery and immediately distilled.
4. The water in the direct-fire stills should be heated almost to boiling before the flowers are charged into the retort.
5. Distillation must proceed smoothly, uniformly, and quickly and must be carefully supervised.
6. The fractions must be sharply cut off.
7. Condensation *must* be efficient.
8. The condensers—all parts of the still—must be immaculate.

The "extra" Ylang-Ylang oil comes out in the first hour. "First" comes off in the first 2 1/2 hours. "Second" comes off in the first 3 to 4 hours. "Third" comes off after this. Total time for this is up to 14 hours. There are other ways to do the distillation which take longer and depends upon distillation time and heat produced.

Ylang-Ylang oil is very complex with many constituents including Methyl Benzoate, Methyl Salicylate, Eugenol, Cresol, Linaloöl, Geraniol, and Terpenes such as Pinene, Cadinene. The percentages are 33–38% Sesquiterpenes, 52–64% alcohols and Esters, and 3% Phenols plus Terpenes, Aldehydes, and Ketones. Ylang-Ylang oil is also produced by extraction with ether, which forms a concrète and absolute.

*General Uses:* In general, Ylang-Ylang oil is an aphrodisiac, nerve tonic, euphoric, cardiotonic, generally sedative, eases depression, eases frigidity and impotence, used in bath and body oil and other body care products for oily skin, and to soothe anger and ease physical pain.

*Properties, Indications, & Uses: Cananga odorata* forma *genuina*: Antispasmodic, creates a feeling of equilibrium in the body, sexual tonic, and used by diabetics to balance the system.

*Indicated for:* Arterial hypertension, sexual weakness, and, particularly, frigidity. The "second' and "thirds" are used as an antispasmodic, anti-inflammatory, antiparasite, for congestion of the pelvic area and abdomen, and skin conditions including itches, scabs, and mange.

Cananga oil specifically is used as a sexual tonic, especially frigidity and balancing.

## Zdravetz (*Geranium macrorrhizum*)

*Family:* Geraniaceae

The name means "health" and the herb is used medicinally. The oil which is distilled in Bulgaria has some use in perfumery and soap making. —from Jeanne Rose *Herbal Body Book,* 1976.

*Habitat & Growth:* A low growing shrub found mostly in Bulgaria.

*Scent:* A masculine, hormonal, and herbaceous odor.

*Components:* Up to 16% Sesquiterpenes, up 50% Sesquiterpinones, particularly Germacrone.

*Properties, Indications, & Uses:* Mainly antitumor. Indicated for certain cancers and pathology in the respiratory and reproductive system.

*Uses:* Mainly externally in massage for these the above conditions. Can be inhaled as well.

*Contraindications:* Not to be used on babies, children, and pregnant women.

Many thanks to Marianne Griffith who helped with the scent descriptions. She continually drafted the scents, and when I reminded her to "Waft, not draft," she said, "I have a big nose, I can handle it!"

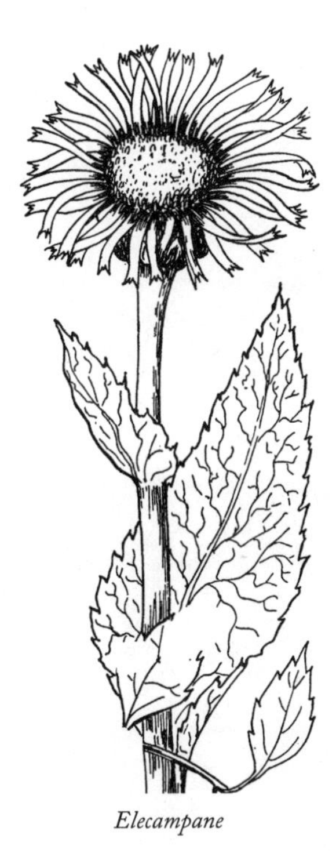

*Elecampane*

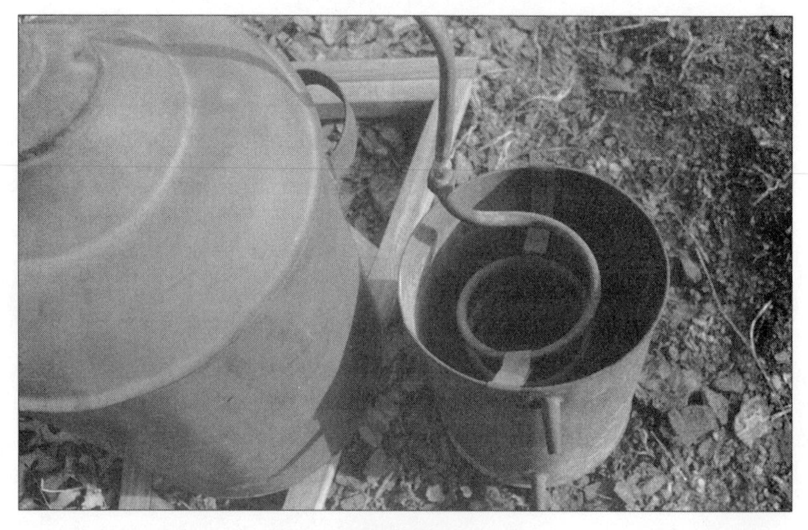

*Old spirit still*

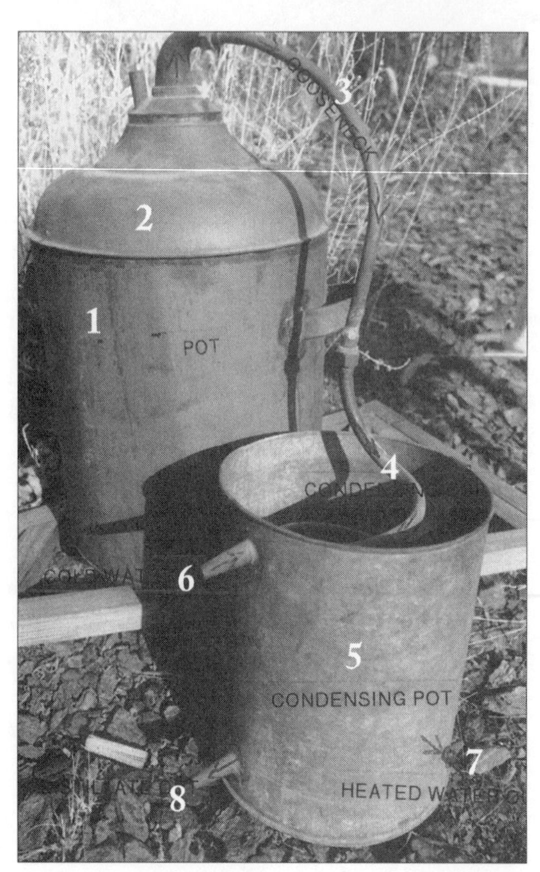


*Spirit still with names of parts*

1 *Pot*
2 *head*
3 *gooseneck*
4 *condensing coil*
5 *condensor*
6 *cold water in*
7 *heated water out*
8 *hydrosol and essential oil out*

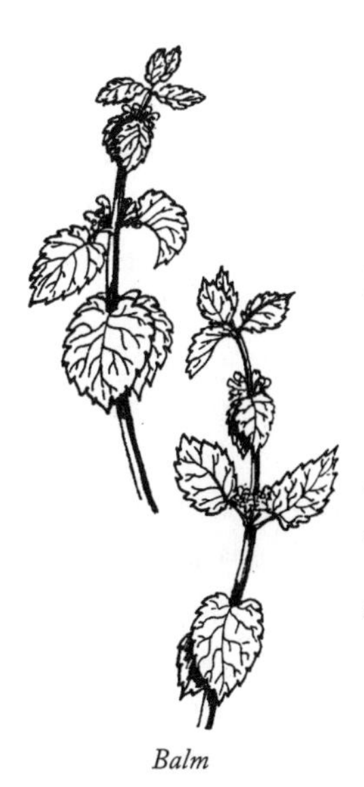

*Balm*

# SIX

# Hydrosols

## The Real Product of Distillation

Hydrosols are the real aromatherapy. They can also be considered the homeopathy of aromatherapy; as herbs are to homeopathy, so are essential oils to hydrosols. Hydrosols represent the true synergy of herbalism and aromatherapy, Hydrosols are the pure natural water that is produced during the distillation process. When plants or flowers are put into the still or distillation tank, they are subjected to either boiling water, or steam or both. The steam hits the plant, softens the scent cells and the essential oil that is contained within is released as a vapor. This essential oil vapor mixes with the steam and is only separated again as the steam cools in the condensing tank. As the steam cools, the essential oil molecules separate from the steam (now as cooled water) and float to the surface because of the specific gravity difference between the essential oil and water, leaving two separate layers in the collecting receiver. The upper layer is the essential oil which floats on the water (except for the very few of them which sink) and the water, now is called the hydrosol, or sometimes, the hydrolat.

Hydrosols from flowers are called flower waters or flower hydrosols and hydrosols from herbs are called herbal hydrosols. In practice they are called as an example, Orange flower water, Geranium hydrosol, Melissa hydrosol.

It is important to remember that the essential oil which is composed of many different chemical molecules is usually lighter than water, therefore floating upon it, and that it is not oily or fatty like a vegetable or animal oil. Essential oils contain no fatty molecules; however, essential oils can be diluted and mix easily with any fatty substance or can be dissolved in alcohol. These, the fatty oils or alcohol, are called carrier substances.

These hydrosols are not simply misters, nor are they water to which droplets of essential oil have been added. They are a separate and natural product of the distillation process and can be termed 100% distilled non-alcoholic distillates. They can not be manufactured synthetically in the laboratory. A hydrosol has to have been produced during the distillation process, preferably using a copper condenser.

In his book *Medical Aromatherapy,* Kurt Schnaubelt's book has commented on hydrosols. "Aromatic hydrosols are the product of steam distillation process and contain the water soluble, volatile components of the plant that often gives them a fragrance quite like the essential oil but not as strong. Their composition is different from that of the essential oil: richer in water-compatible components and free of very lipophilic substances such as terpene hydrocarbons. This means highly tolerable, antiinflammative, and antiseptic substances are found in aromatic hydrosols." [1]

Hydrosol is the other product of distillation that occurs when plants are water or steam-distilled to release the fragrance, the essential oil. The term is a combination of hydro (water) and sol (solution)—a natural water solution that contains some water-soluble microdrops of essential oil as well as water-soluble plant components. The microdrops of essential oil give the hydrosol its scent and taste. The plant components give the hydrosol its herbal or floral therapy. Hydrosols are 100% distilled, used at full strength exactly as they are, straight from the still. They can also be diluted with water or in tea and used as a therapeutic drink (1 tablespoon/liter or 1–3).

[1] Kurt Schnaubelt, *Medical Aromatherapy.* (Berkeley, CA: North Atlantic Books, 1999).

## The Aromatic Plant Project

Now that you know why you want them, it is nice to know that these miracle waters are produced in this country from plants grown right here. A special project has been initiated in the United States allowing us to have the finest and freshest products available. Perhaps more important, this program creates an example, albeit on a small scale, for society as a whole, of right livelihood, respect for the environment, increasing the knowledge of therapeutic plants and sustainable agriculture. *The Aromatic Plant Project* was founded in 1990 in the United States to encourage the local growing and distillation of true essential oil plants for the production of hydrosols and, in some cases, essential oils.

This project began with a journey into the California wine country. Armed with a few bottles of different types of Lavender essential oil, I introduced some wine growers to the variations in quality and scent in essential oils in the same manner that wine makers discuss the different fragrances and tastes of wines. As the wine makers pulled out bottles of wine from different vintages years representing grapes from different fields and different elevations, I too pulled out my bottles of Lavender representing different sources and different distillations. As the fragrances and tastes of the wines varies with topology, so did the Lavender essential oils.

The grape growers and wine makers understood the concept of *terroir*—different elevations, soil types, amount of rainfall, slope changes—and how these conditions, the topology, can affect the taste and scent of a wine. They understood that terroir has much the same effect on essential oil plants.

Initially, they were excited about the possibility of growing a crop of essential oil plants alongside the valuable wine grapes. These could be harvested in the off-season, providing additional income from the sale of hydrosols and essential oils. In addition, they knew that essential oil plants would discourage insect and fungal infestations along the roots and leaves of their valuable wine grapes. Esthetically, the herbs and flowers from the essential oil plants would provide a visual treat for tourists who came to visit the vineyards.

It has not been the grape grower and wine maker, however, who has become the prime grower of essential oil plants for hydrosols. Rather it has been the owners of small amounts of acreage who saw the potential of keeping the land out of the hands of developers and who wished to cultivate and plant it with organically grown plants for the production of essential oils and hydrosols.

The concept for an association was formed. I began to write letters to a variety of growers and distillers and then named it *the Association of the Aromatic Plant Project* (APP), which is a nonprofit educational organization. The APP only accepts growers who use organic growing methods. It provides literature and lists of growers and distillers to members, consumers and interested parties, and can be reached by phone (see Chapter 9, p. 211). The growers have been planting particular strains of Lavender (*Lavandula* spp.), Pelargoniums (so-called Rose Geranium), Lemon Verbena (*Aloysia triphylla*), Lemon Balm (*Melissa*) and other plants. Plants are chosen on the basis of lab analysis that when distilled yield a high quality essential oil and hydrosol whose type and quantity of chemical components are considered therapeutic.

For example, in the case of the Lavender species, it has been determined that a quality Lavandin essential oil contains 40%+ linaloöl, 22%+ of the ester linalyl acetate, little to *no camphor,* under 8% cineol and—for California grown Lavenders—up to 8% borneol. Borneol is accepted in this case in Lavender, because it is considered to be an immune stimulant. This particular essential oil is very high in the soothing linalyl acetate, sedating linaloöl, and immune–stimulating borneol. In California, a fine-smelling, soft, and fragrant essential oil is produced with all these particular qualities from *Lavandula x intermedia* cv Grosso, CT linaloöl/borneol. This special plant is only available from two select nurseries on the west coast of the United States. In contrast, Lavender hydrosol made from 'landscape' Lavenders has cineole (as in Eucalyptus) which is a mucolytic for the respiratory system and smells like Eucalyptus oil, but does not have the necessary Lavender qualities of soothing and sedation.

Distillers, the people who distill the plants, of *The Aromatic Plant Project* are competent, knowledgeable people who have many years of training in the production of fine-quality essential oils and hydrosols. Of course, when a fine quality essential oil plant is produced, then the hydrosol, if perfectly distilled, can be of high quality as well.

Distillers must choose ahead of time whether to distill for the hydrosol or the essential oil. Good quality hydrosols are very slowly, expertly distilled with low heat, where the temperature is very low, maybe 102 degrees centigrade. The problem, of course, is that whenever people think about distillation, they're thinking about essential oils. You have to choose ahead of time whether you're going to distill for the essential oil or the hydrosol. When you distill for a hydrosol, you use plants that have just been harvested. You can get both essential oil and hydrosol of *quality* when you are distilling for the hydrosol. You cannot get *quantity* of essential oil if you're distilling for the hydrosol. When you distill for essential oil, you let plants air-dry for a day or two before distillation, this way more plant material can be packed into the still, thus resulting in more essential oil. You cannot get *quality* of hydrosol if you're really just distilling for the essential oil, and this is the reason: distillation for the essential oil starts with air-dried plants; whereas distillation for the hydrosol starts with freshly picked plants with their moisture intact. With my personal distillation equipment, the pot is about 5 feet tall, and about 6 feet around. It holds up to 5–20 lbs. of plant material, depending on if it is wet or dry.

When you pick the Lavender or the Lemon Balm or the Lemon Verbena, you want to dry it for a day or two for *the essential oil,* because you want to reduce and compact the volume—you want to put as much plant material into the pot as possible to reduce the volume and increase the weight of the plant. In the case of Lemon Verbena and Lemon Balm, which produce only microscopic amounts of essential oil, we distill only for the hydrosol. For it is only with cohobation that any essential oil can be produced from these two plants and this process (cohobation) ruins the hydrosol. The process of cohobation repeatedly returns the hydrosol to the distillation chamber to concentrate the essential oil.

In the case of a traditional distillation of Lemon Verbena and Lemon Balm, the hydrosol itself, has contained within it all the essential oil of the plant, its water soluble plant properties and therefore, all the therapeutic quality. Lemon Verbena and Lemon Balm oil are potent viricides and can be used as a spray application of the hydrosol to herpes or genital warts.

The marketers of *The Aromatic Plant Project* are visionaries who see the future of aromatherapy, and it is with the hydrosols and the products made from them, as well as with quality essential oils. All things considered, however, it is ultimately you—the consumer—who will determine the value of these products. Your buying dollar becomes the ultimate endorsement and ensures that this project can continue. It is our hope that with the education and support of publications like *The Aromatic Thymes*, the public will become thoroughly educated about the usefulness and value of these products and support their continued production.

## Hydrosols—A Multitude of Uses

The beauty and pleasure of simply spritzing yourself—face, hair, body, and clothes—with the gentle fragrance

- Cool a hot flash.
- Soothe a sunburn.
- Soothe a pet's hot spots.
- Clean the air.
- Freshen the bathroom.
- Keep in the entryway to freshen the air before guests arrive.

*Hygiene*

- Disinfect your hands.
- Make your own wet wipes—spray on a tissue or damp cloth and use. Great for you, your pets, your baby. Good for dirty faces, hands, and bottoms.
- Use for a healing sitz bath.

*Travel*

- Refresh the air during travel—car, hotel room, airplane. Cleanse that recycled air.
- Hydrosols act as air-borne viricides.

*Beverages*

- Add 1 teaspoon in 6 to 8 oz. water—distilled,

mineral, or otherwise. Ice cubes and sweetener optional.
- Add a splash to a glass of white wine or champagne.

*Laundry*
- Spray in the dryer before adding clothes and then directly on the clothes.
- Spray on clothes during ironing.

*Fine dining*
- Spray on cloth napkins and tablecloth to refresh the scent already used in the dryer and while ironing.
- Place bowls of hydrosol with flowers floating in them in the centerpiece to scent the room.
- Serve smaller finger bowls of the same on silver trays at the end of the meal for guests to clean their hands.

*Beauty and skin care*
- Spritz on fingernails to encourage healthy growth of nails.
- Spritz on face to set makeup.
- Spritz on hair and scrunch to refresh and scent hairdo.
- Add to cream and lotion products to increase their efficacy.
- Add a few cups to the bath.

*Note:* Fresh hydrosol, that has been cleanly distilled is pure and free of bacteria. It should be stored in the refrigerator, used within the year it is distilled, and thrown out at the next distillation, which will be when the plants are mature again. Old hydrosol can also be used in the bath. Put old hydrosols in your room fountains or anything that circulates water. Fresh, pure hydrosols do not need preservation, if care is taken during the distillation. Do not let people run their fingers through the distillate as it comes from the still. It should be dripped directly into a sterile container, than sealed and refrigerated.

**Uses of Floral Hydrosols**

| Floral Hydrosols (Waters) | External/Skin Care | Mental Care | Internal/Culinary |
|---|---|---|---|
| *Artemisia arborescens* | damaged skin, anti-spasmodic, anti-inflammatory, eases joint pain | mildly calming, strongly energizing | none/none |
| Chamomile, German | anti-inflammatory for soothing, irritated skin | emotionally calming | calming tea/none |
| Chamomile, Roman | anti-inflammatory for dry, inflamed, sensitive skin | psychic soother | calming tea/none |
| Cornflower | eyewash, skin toner, dry or mature skin, bruising | hot flashes, relaxing | calming tea/none |
| Goldenrod | anti-inflammatory, astringent | relaxing | possible diuretic/none |
| Jasmine | true hydrosol does not exist | energizing | none/none |
| Lavender, True | gentle, balancing, cooling, all skin types, universal toner, esp., for oily or impure skin, for sensitive skin, cools burned skin, hydrating, balancing, bathing | eases mental stress, reduces mental fatigue, for jet lag | relaxing, revitalizing/can be added to mineral water or all dessert foods |

**Uses of Floral Hydrosols, cont.**

| Floral Hydrosols (Waters) | External/Skin Care | Mental Care | Internal/Culinary |
|---|---|---|---|
| Lavandin | bathing, toner | relaxing, revitalizing | cleansing/add to mineral water |
| Lavandin CT, Borneol | acne or herpes | stimulating | immune stimulating/add to desserts or jellies |
| Linden | all types of skin care, spray for shingles | calming., relaxing, sedative, baby care, dreaming | relaxing/savory and sweet dishes |
| Orange Blossom | hydrating to dry skin, for bathing, gentle for babies | aphrodisiac, uplifting | 1 tsp. in cup of coffee eliminates jitters/desserts |
| Rose | toner for all skin types, aftershave, after bath splash | aphrodisiac, eases nervousness and mental strain | ease heart pains/add to desserts or jellies, yummy |
| Yarrow flowers | anti-inflammatory, antiseptic, acne, damaged skin, cellulite | energetic, spiritual healing, auric or aura protection | none/none |

Floral waters are hydrosols made from flowers.

### Uses of Herbal Hydrosols

| Herbal Hydrosols | External/Skin Care | Mental Care | Internal/Culinary |
|---|---|---|---|
| Basil | stimulating/hair loss | calming, a fiery feeling | calms nausea/tasty on vegetables and pastas; digestive, slight licorice taste |
| Bay Laurel | toning, aftershave, man's skin & scent | uplifting | digestive/good with meat foods, sprinkle on steamed veggies |
| Black Spruce | relieves pain, male skin care, relieves itching | for stress | tonic/resinous taste |
| Carrot tops | anti-inflammatory, soothes irritated, itchy, dry skin | none | Woman's tea/imparts an earthy, sweet aroma and flavor |
| Clary Sage | astringent, oily skin | PMS hot flashes, drug withdrawl, energetic | for menstrual problems/on sweets and most desserts |
| Eucalyptus | helpful for blemishes & acne, regenerative | purifies the air | respiratory/none |
| Everlast (Helichrysum) | heals and soothes irritations, depleted and inflamed conditions, helpful in reducing scarring when used on fresh wounds | detoxifying, soothes the heart | liver and gall bladder healer/can be added to mineral water or wherever a honey scent is desired |

**Uses of Herbal Hydrosols, cont.**

| Herbal Hydrosols | External/Skin Care | Mental Care | Internal/Culinary |
|---|---|---|---|
| Fennel seed | antiseptic, eye cleansing, skin soother | comforting | digestive, eases stomachache, may promote lactation/tasty licorice flavor |
| Juniper berry | detox, stimulates circulation, oily skin, reduces puffiness | energetic | diuretic, good study tea/great in marinades, detox |
| Lemon Balm (Melissa) | herpes, for bathing | calming, sedating, insomnia, mental stress | viricide in water/for cooking lamb, in fruit punch |
| Lemon Verbena | revitalizing to normal skin types, balancing | stimulating | as a sleep aid/delicious in tea |
| Linden | very soothing | relaxing, relieves anxiety, depression, insomnia, euphoric | as a sleep aid/in mineral water |
| Myrtle | external eye wash, all over skin care, irritations | relieves fatigue, refreshing, reviving | spray for sore throats and coughs/ some use in cooking on meats, fish |
| Oregano | strong antiseptic, antibacterial, douche or sitz bath, anti-viral, anti-fungal | none | daily tonic drink/good beverage, ood taste |

**Uses of Herbal Hydrosols, cont.**

| Herbal Hydrosols | External/Skin Care | Mental Care | Internal/Culinary |
|---|---|---|---|
| Peppermint | relieves itching, redness, inflammation and acne, cooling, for bathing | uplifting, energizing, cooling, for hot flashes | taken by itself to soothe digestion/on all mint-loving foods |
| Rose Geranium | for bathing, cellular regenerative, balances oil glands oily or dry skin, cleans up doggy odor | stimulates adrenal cortex, antidepressant, cooling, for hot flashes | woman hormonal imbalance/water, jellies, fruit desserts |
| Rosemary | revitalizes skin, for bathing | restores energy, alertness, for tired feet | internal stimulant/meat dishes, sprinkle on steamed veggies |
| Thyme | acne, dermatitis, eczema, insect bites | stimulating, increases circulation, revitalizes | antiseptic, digestive/for lamb or non-sweet cookies, for veggies |
| Witch Hazel | anti-inflammatory, antiseptic, antifungal, spray for varicose veins and hemorrhoids | none | cleansing/mildly tasty |

Herbal hydrosols are hydrosols made from herbs and their green parts.

## A Double Distillation — Stainless vs. Copper

Over the Memorial Day weekend in 1998, I met with 15 students and another distiller to test the quality of distilling in stainless steel versus distillation in a traditional copper pot still. We met early on a Saturday morning and discussed the various ways to harvest plants. As we walked through the Rose Geranium (*Pelargonium graveolens*) field we discussed botany, terroir and harvest techniques. Several different groups separated—some harvesting with a simple knife, others with clippers and others with a two-handed method; using one hand to hold the top of the plant and the other to slice across the plant with a knife.

Rose Geranium should be two years old before it is harvested. The younger plants produce bright, spritely-smelling essential oils and hydrosols, while the older plants produce a more mature smelling essential oil and a rich, fragrant hydrosol. These plants were two years old and had not been over-watered. Therefore, they had small, tight leaves that were not overly fat or juicy, but covered with essential oil glands. The top third of the plant is taken; particularly the leaves, leaving behind the fat stalks. The plant should be in full flower. Our Rose Geranium was mature, full of flowers and very fragrant. We harvested the top third and went back to the still area where the two stills were set up. To produce quality hydrosols, we start with freshly cut plants that have not been allowed to dry out.

One distiller had a vertical stainless steel still that will hold about 150 pounds of fresh Lavender or Rose Geranium plant. The copper still holds about 25 pounds of fresh material. Both stills were loaded and within three hours we had completed the distillation.

*Stainless Steel*
Steam distillation
50 pounds of plant material
Steam from a separate steam generator
Plants in pot with steam
Stainless steel vertical condensing pipes

Produced 5 gallons of hydrosol
• green-smelling with a distinct composty note, not acceptable

*Copper*
Water/steam distillation
10 pounds of plant material
5 gallons of water in pot
Plants in pot held above water
via a screen
Copper condensing coil

Produced 2 gallons of hydrosol
- sweet-smelling, immediately acceptable

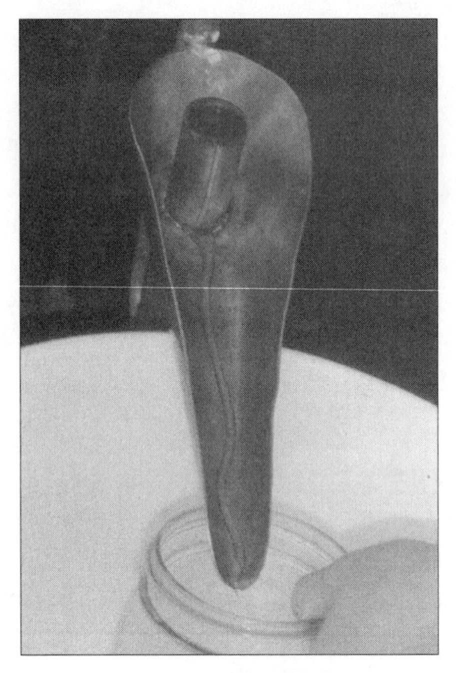

*Here comes the hydrosol*

**Hydrosol Still**

| | |
|---|---|
| Size | 3–5 Gallon Boiler, ½ to 3 lbs. of plant material, (e.g. ½ lb. of Lemon Verbena, 1–1½ lbs. of Chamomile, etc.<br>Yields 1 to 5 lbs. of HYDROSOL |
| Heat | Kitchen stove, Gas or Electric |
| Cooling | Water from sink faucet. Return water to sink drain. |
| Storage | In single shipping box. Lid with cooling devices and all accessories fits inside of boiler for storage when not in use. |
| Parts and Repairs | Available from CH-Imports. |
| Price | $325 for complete still. All sink connections and hoses included. |
| Terms | $175 with orders. Balance COD, FOB Greensboro, NC. |
| Delivery | 3–4 weeks via UPS ground transportation. |
| Quantity | Discounts available for multiple units to resellers. |
| Order From | CH-Imports, Ltd.<br>P.O. Box 18411<br>Greensboro, NC 27419<br>Phone (336) 282-9734, Fax (336) 288-3375 |

## Hydrosol Still

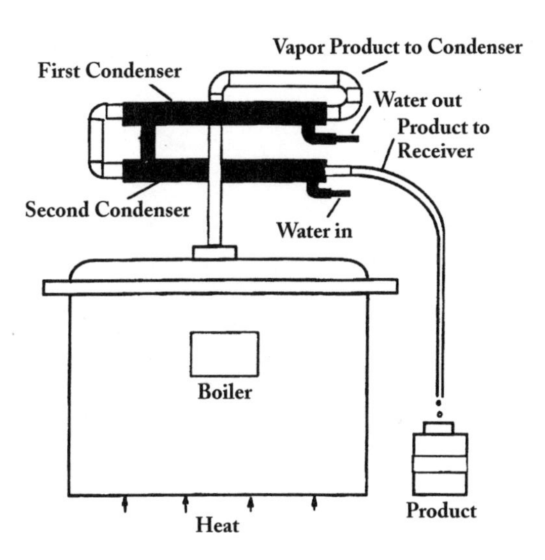

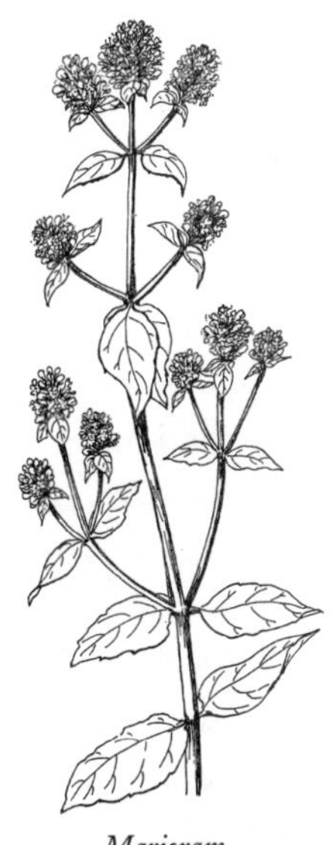
*Marjoram*

SEVEN

# A Variety of Plant Essays

There is so much to know regarding aromatherapy and particularly the specific botany of each plant and its essential oil. These essays attempt to clear up some of the mystery about some plants and their essential oils. You should also look at the various aromatherapy magazines that are now available. Some of them produce a plant essential oil profile in each issue. This information should include the common name of the oil, the Latin binomial and botanical family name, countries of origin, description of the plant, habitat and growth, portion of the plant used in distillation, extraction method and yield, physical characteristics of the oil, chemical components, historical facts, properties and *how* the EO is used, physical and emotional uses, key use and safety data and precautions.

## The Evergreens and Their Similars

Cedar, Cypress, Juniper, Fir, Pine & Spruce are all Evergreen trees whose bark, needles and sometimes wood and cones produce essential oil. Their oils are commonly considered useful for respiratory care and for care of the upper, airy parts of the body and it is often said that this is because they come from tall trees whose leaves or needles are touching the sky. They have refreshing, mind-clearing fragrances that are strong yet somehow translucent. When one begins to take a closer look at the Evergreen plants and their essential oils, confusion quickly ensues! As we talk about the plants and their oils individually, you will become increasingly aware of the importance of being educated and informed as an aromatherapy practitioner as well as the importance of purchasing your essential oils from a source that is educated and informed and willing to share information with you. I have tried to make this as clear and understandable as possible, yet, as I speak individually about the oils, please remember, you are not the only one who is confused! I highly recommend that you perform your own research. Collect the Evergreen plants. Compare the differences in their leaves, barks and cones. Collect the Evergreen essential oils from various sources and be sure to use the Latin name when labeling the plants and purchasing the essential oils. Compare the fragrances and make a journal of the information you find. A project such as this will help you at least to *understand* the confusion, if not to clear some of it up.

We have divided the Evergreen trees into six parts and given the general common name to each part:

**Family Pinaceae**

I. *Pinus* also known as Pine
II. *Picea* also known as Spruce
III. *Abies* also known as Fir
*Tsuga* also known as Hemlock
*Pseudotsuga* also known as False Hemlock
IV. *Cedrus* also known as True Cedar

**Family Cupressaceae**

V. *Cupressus* also known as Cypress, Thuja and Chamaecyparis
VI. *Juniperus* also known as Juniper

## THE PINACEAE FAMILY

In Group I we find the Pinus species in the family *Pinaceae.* There is only confusion among users of essential oils in that the family *Pinaceae* includes a variety of trees with interchangeable common names. These names include: Firs, Spruces, Pines, Cedars, the

Turpentine pines, and other plants that are often considered Cypress, Juniper or Spruce. Briefly, family *Pinaceae* includes: Pinus species; *Picea* species, such as *Picea abies* (Norway Spruce) and *Picea mariana* (Black Spruce); *Tsuga canadensis* and *T. heterophylla,* the Hemlocks; *Pseudotsuga douglasii* (Douglas Fir); and the *Abies* species, such as *Abies sibirica* (Siberian Fir); and true Cedar species, such as, *Cedrus atlantica* (Atlas Cedarwood).

## **Group I. Pinus** (Pines)

Trees of the Genus *Pinus* have leaves that are persistent and of two kinds, the primary ones are linear or scale-like, and deciduous. The secondary ones form the ordinary foliage and are narrowly linear (needle-like), arising from the axils of the primary leaves in bunches of 1-5 leaf clusters enclosed at the base in a membranous sheath.

Mainly the trees that produce the essential oils that are called Pine oil are *Pinus mugo* (Dwarf Pine), *Pinus palustris* (Long Leaf Pine) and *Pinus sylvestris* (Scotch Pine).

*Pinus mugo* (Dwarf Pine Needle). Is harvested in the Swiss Alps. It is sturdy and shrub-like and is protected by the Swiss government and is harvested according to particular rules only at certain elevations. This oil has a particularly pungent odor reminiscent of both a bark and needle oil and in fact entire branches including the needles are finely chopped up and thrown into the still for the essential oil. This combination of bark and needle make up an oil that is both airy and grounding.

Components of Dwarf Pine Needle oil include l-α Pinene, β-Pinene, l-Limonene, Sesquiterpenes, Pumiliol, etc.

In Europe, this plant is used for diseases of the skin and scalp and particularly at healing spas where it is inhaled for ailments of the respiratory organs, including pleurisy and tuberculosis. This is a powerful adjunct in the therapies for all sorts of ear, nose, throat and lung disorders.

*Pinus pinaster* (Maritime Pine). Contains Mono and Sesquiterpenes. It is a powerful antiseptic used to disinfect the air locally. Good for chronic bronchitis, chronic cystitis, and anti-inflammatory for the lungs. Can be used externally in massage blends for rheumatism or aching joints.

A chemotype of *Pinus pinaster* contains large quantities of terebenthine which is composed of 62% α-Pinene and 27% β-Pinene. This oleo-resin is used as a powerful expectorant, antiseptic, and to oxygenate the air. Indicated for infections of the respiratory system. In hot water for steam inhaling treatments. Mainly used as an aerosol treatment with possible allergies if used externally.

*Pinus palustris* (Long Leaf Pine, Turpentine) (See Terebinth). A tall, evergreen, up to 150 feet with attractive, reddish-brown, deeply fissured bark with long, stiff needles that grow in pairs. Is used mainly for the distillation of American gum sprits of Turpentine. This is a tall, evergreen tree native to the Southeast United States.

The main component is Terpineol.

It has been considered a powerful antiseptic spray and disinfectant, especially in veterinary medicine. It has mainly been used externally as a massage for arthritis, muscular aches and pains and stiffness, and natural Turpentine has often been inhaled for asthma and bronchitis. This has been much used in commercial industry to manufacture paint, but has now been largely replaced by synthetic Pine oil (synth. Turpentine).

*Pinus sylvestris* (Scotch Pine or Norway Pine). A tall, evergreen, up to 150 feet with attractive, reddish-brown, deeply fissured bark with long, stiff needles that grow in pairs. Essential oil is produced mainly in the Baltic states. The components are greatly influenced by geographical origin and consist mainly of Monoterpenes, Pinene, some Limonene.

*Pinus sylvestris* is considered to have hormone-like, cortisone-like qualities. It is indicated for convalescence, inhaled for bronchitis, sinusitis and asthma and is used to tone the respiratory system, balance the hypothalamic/pancreas axis as well as the HPA (hypothalamus-pituitary-adrenal). It is a hypertensive, tonic stimulant.

## **Group II. Picea** (Spruce)

The second group of trees of the *Pinaceae* family are generally called Spruce trees. Some Spruce trees also have the common name of Fir.

Genera *Picea* leaves are linear, often obtuse or emarginate base of leaves persistent on the branches. The leaves are sessile, 4-sided, or flattened and stomatiferous.

Spruce trees which are of the Genera *Picea,* are conical trees with linear short 4-sided leaves spreading in all directions, jointed at the base to a short persistent sterigmata, on which they are sessile, falling away in drying, the bare twigs appearing covered with low, truncate projections. The leaf buds are scaly. Cones are ovid to oblong, obtuse, pendulous, their scales numerous, spirally arranged, thin, obtuse, persistent.

Black Spruce *(Picea mariana).* The essential oil has much value in the respiratory system. The components include 55% Monoterpenes, including Camphene, α-Pinene, γ-Bornyl acetate, etc. The properties are hormone-like, possibly stimulating the thymus gland and with cortisone-like properties that affect the HPA axis.

*Picea mariana* (Black Spruce) grows in Quebec, Canada. Components also include Monoterpenes, including α-Pinene and γ-3-Carene, and Sesquiterpenes. Indicated for bronchitis; internal parasites and an antifungal for candida; prostatitis; solar plexus spasms; asthenic conditions; excellent for sudden fatigue or exhaustion. A general tonic for the entire system and indicated as well for excessive thyroid function. Possibly this oil is extremely valuable inhaled for asthmatics who take cortico-steroids.

*Picea alba* (White Spruce). Different chemical components from Black Spruce. Both White and Black Spruce contain Tricylene. Uses of these oils are: included in "Cedar" blends for technical laboratory preparations, room sprays, deodorants.

*Picea excelsa* (Norway Spruce). Young twigs and leaves are steam distilled in the Tyrol valley. Chemical composition is mainly Pinene, Phellandrene and Dipentene, etc. Norway Spruce has a very fragrant odor and it is used in all sorts of Pine-scented compositions, bath salts, room sprays, etc.

## **Group III. Abies** (Fir), **Tsuga** (Hemlock), **Pseudotsuga** (Mock Hemlock)

In Group III we find the common name of Firs from the Family *Pinaceae* and these include a variety of trees called Fir.

The Firs are distributed worldwide and are coniferous trees with pyramid shapes. The essential oil is generally steam distilled from small twigs and needles.

***Tsuga (Hemlocks).***

Leaves of the *genera Tsuga* are stalked, flattened and stomatiferous below, or angular, often appearing 2-ranked.

Hemlocks include *Tsuga canadensis* (Eastern Hemlock), *Tsuga heterophylla* (the Western Hemlock also called Gray Fir or Alaskan Pine) and sometimes the Black Spruce and White Spruce.

These trees have slender horizontal or drooping branches, flat narrowly linear scattered short-petioled leaves, spreading and appearing 2-ranked, jointed to very short sterigmata and falling away in drying. The leaf-buds are scaly. Hemlocks are widely known in North America. These trees are tall evergreens with horizontal branches and finely toothed leaves. The young branches and leaves are steam distilled. Production is normally in the Northeastern part of United States.

*Tsuga canadensis* is native to the West coast. Twigs and needles are S-D. It is an antiseptic, astringent, diuretic. The bark tea is used for diarrhea, cystitis, colitis, uterine prolapse. A bark extract is used in tanning. It is non-toxic, non-irritating and non-sensitizing. The EO can be inhaled for asthma, coughs, bronchitis, colds and flu. Externally it is used for muscular aches and rheumatism. It blends well with Pine, Oakmoss, Cedars, benzoin, Lavender and Rosemary.

***Pseudotsuga or False Hemlock.***

The base of the leaves of trees of the Pseudotsuga genera are not persistent on the branches. The leaves often appear 2-ranked, are stalked, flattened, stomatiferous below; winter-buds are pointed, not resinous.

*Pseudotsuga douglasii* (Douglas Fir/*P. menziesii),* a native to the West Coast of the United States and now grown elsewhere. It is a tall, attractive evergreen Fir tree, much used in the Christmas tree industry. If you diffuse this oil in late November and early December you are sure to inspire the "Christmas spirit" in even the most grouchy of scrooges! It is a wonderful oil to wake up to at that particular time of year.

The leaves are steam distilled to create the essential oil whose components vary considerably. The French oil contains large quantities of β-Pinene and smaller amounts of Citronellyl acetate and β-Phellandrene.

Douglas Fir essential oil is strongly antiseptic and indicated for respiratory infections. It can be used as a local disinfectant. This is one of the most lemon-scented of the Firs, with a powerful sweet, fresh, refreshing odor, well-liked as a room refresher or scent in soap blends.

*Pseudotsuga taxifolia.* Turpentine oil from *Pseudotsuga taxifolia* is actually an oleo-resin produced in the crevices of the tree trunk. On S-D it produces up to 35% the volatile oil, which is composed of up to 55 % l-α-Pinene, etc. Turpentine is used commercially in technical preparations.

***Abies (True Firs).***

The base of the leaves of this group of trees is not persistent on the branches. The leaves often appear 2-ranked but are actually spirally arranged. The leaves are sessile, flattened and often grooved on the upper side or quadrangular, rarely stomatiferous above and on the upper fertile branches they are often crowded. The winter-buds are obtuse and resinous.

*Pseudotsuga taxifolia* and *Abies balsamea* (Canada Balsam Fir). Turpentine oil is produced from both *Pseudotsuga taxifolia* and *Abies balsamea.* This product is also a true turpentine because it consists of both resin and volatile oil. Component is principally l-α-Pinene.

*Abies balsamea* (Balsam Fir). It contains up to 90% Monoterpenes. It is antiseptic and antispasmodic and is inhaled for the respiratory system.

*Abies siberica* (Siberian Fir). Widely grown in Russia. Its chief constituent, 40%, is l-Bornyl acetate. Its properties are antispasmodic and used for bronchitis and asthma.

*Abies alba* (White Fir). Contains 95% Monoterpenes. It is an antiseptic; inhaled for respiratory problems. In addition, *Abies alba* produces a cone oil with a very pleasant balsamic odor consisting chiefly of l-Limonene and used as an adjunct in all Pine needle scents.

*Abies sachalinensis* and *Abies mariana* . Called Pine needle oils, but are actually Firs. They are commonly called Japanese Pine Needle. They contain mainly l-Limonene and Sesquiterpenes. Primarily used for respiratory inhalations and for scenting of soap.

## **Group IV. Cedrus** (True Cedars)

The *Cedrus genera* has needles arranged singly on growing shoots in tufts often called "whorls". There are often 10-20 needles arranged in one tuft. The Cedrus genera have upright cones like the *Abies,* but the cones disintegrate after two years.

Cedar *needle* oils are generally used externally, well diluted for skin conditions and dandruff, fungal infections and hair loss, and inhaled in blends for the respiratory system. Cedar oils are contraindicated for people who are prone to high blood pressure and heart problems and should be avoided by people with sensitive skin.

**Confusion in the Use of the Name Cedar**

Cedar is a common name used for a variety of plants from both family *Pinaceae* and family *Cupressaceæ.* Here we encounter the confusion that common names create. There are many types of Cedar trees: true Cedars from the *Genus Cedrus* and other trees which are actually from other Genera, yet have the common name of Cedar. True Cedar, of the *Genera Cedrus*, is from the *Pinaceae* family. There are some trees from the *Cupressaceæ* family which are also called Cedars, but when you look at their Latin binomials you will see that they are Junipers or Thujas. True Cedars from family *Pinaceæ* include Atlas Cedarwood, Deodar Cedarwood and Lebanon Cedarwood. From family *Cupressaceæ*: Port Orford Cedar, Hinoki Cedar, Virginia Cedar, Texas Cedar, and others from the Juniper clan of this group of trees. Remember, the trees called Cedar from the *Cupressaceæ* family are *not* true Cedars. So I recommend, again, call your essential oils by their Latin binomial. This way, you will know for sure from which plant your oil comes.

Another point to be aware of when using Cedar oils is whether you are using the oil of the *leaf* or the *wood.* Awareness of the part of the plant the oil is coming from is just as important as awareness of *which* Cedar the oil is coming from. If an oil is simply labeled Cedar, how are you to know what this oil is and how it can be used safely? All essential oils should be labeled with their Latin binomial, common name, country of origin, and part of the plant used. Although if you look at your collection of essential oils at home or in stores, you will see that this is rarely the case.

*Cedrus atlantica* (Atlas Cedar). Oil from the *wood* of *Cedrus atlantica* from the Pinaceæ family contains up to 80% Sesquiterpenes and

Sesquiterpenols. Its properties are an arterial regenerative and a lymphotonic. It aids in the removal of body fat, and used externally for cellulite and the retention of fluid in the tissue and is indicated for artherosclerosis. Atlas Cedar is a good oil for the medicine chest because it is used for the respiratory system; a drop in a half cup water to gargle for sore throat; or with a few drops of Eucalyptus in a steaming bowl of water to reduce nasal and lung congestion. This would be a good oil to use in a home-made vapor salve, something like "Vicks Vapo-Rub" for relief of lung and nasal congestion. It can be added to shampoos or facial washes to reduce oily secretions. It is also used as a fixative in the perfume industry. This oil is considered to be neurotoxic and abortive so should not be used for children and pregnant women.

*Cedrus deodara* (Himalayan Cedarwood). Himalayan Cedar*wood* from the *Pinaceæ* family contains a quantity of Sesquiterpenes and is very close to Atlas Cedarwood and could be substituted in a number of cases. It regenerates the arterial system, and, like Atlas is a lymphotonic and is indicated for cellulite and water retention. Himalayan Cedarwood is also contraindicated for children and pregnant women because it is considered neurotoxic and abortive.

## THE CUPRESSACEAE FAMILY

The leaves of this family of trees are opposite or whorled, usually scale-like as opposed to needle-like.

### **Group V Thuja** (Arbor Vitae), **Chamaecyparis** ("Cypress"), **Cupressus** (True Cypress)

***Thuja (Arbor Vitae).***

Trees of the *Thuja genera* called Arbor vitae, have internodes about as long as they are broad, often pale below and usually glandular. They have branchlets which are flattened in one plane. They have frond-like foliage.

Included here are: Thuja or "Cedar"leaf oil, *Thuja occidentalis; Thuja plicata* the so-called Western Red "Cedar."

Cypress *(Cupressus spp.). Cupressus spp.* is from the family *Cupressaceae.* Oils from several different plants are sold as 'Cypress.' The oil from a tree of the Thuja genus has a common name of 'Cedar' as well.

Cedar oil from *Thuja occidentalis* is rather toxic and is a skin irritant. *T. occidentalis* foilage are water or steam distilled to produce their essential oil. It has been used to burn off warts, which gives you an idea of just how irritating it is! To use it in this manner, apply a ring of glycerine around the wart, plantar wart or verruca, and apply the oil only to the wart itself. It is fine diluted for use as a disinfectant in household cleaning, but is not an oil to be used in the diffusor or in a massage oil. You can see why it is important that you, as someone using essential oils be educated and why it is important that companies properly label the essential oils they are selling.

The wood of *Thuja plicata* , called "Cedarwood" (on S-D of the wood, a volatile oil is obtained that contains a poisonous ketone—thujopsone). This oil contains thujone and internal use is discouraged as it is considered a convulsant poison. Small amounts of the leaves and bark can be infused for baths and this is especially useful for cleaning the skin of the oils of Poison Oak and Poison Ivy. The scent is refreshing and stimulating. Use of the essential oil in this manner is carefully recommended.

***Chamaecyparis (Cypress).***

This is called a Cypress. It is similar to the Thuja with minute opposite, 4-ranked scale-like leaves. The filaments are broader and shield-shaped.

Hinoki essential oil from *Chamaecyparis obtusa* containing 40% Terpenes and some borneol. It has a camphor odor and is used extensively in Japan in the scenting of soap and in insecticides. It is also immune stimulating and an antibacterial.

The Port Orford Cedar, *Chamaecyparis lawsoniana* containing up to 46% d-α-Pinene, 3% δ-Limonene, 26% δ-borneol, 21% δ-cadinene and 4% cadinol. It is a topical fungicide. Infuse the needles and wood in Olive oil for 12 hours at 140°, paint this on boats to rot-proof the wood.

***Cupressus (True Cypress).***

Trees of the *Genera Cupressus* are the True Cypresses. They have 4-angled branchlets more or less in one plant. The fruit is a cone.

The True Cypresses include Portuguese Cypress from *C. lusitanica;* Guatemala Cypress oil; Monterey Cypress from *C. macrocarpa.*

Lawless uses *Cupressus sempervirens* essential oil in skincare for oily skin, in massage for rheumatism, poor circulation, as an inhalant for asthma and bronchitis and for menstrual and menopausal problems although she does not mention whether this is internal or external use.

*Cupressus sempervirens* (Cypress). A tall evergreen tree native to the Mediterranean containing 45% Monoterpenes and Sesquiterpenes such as 7% Cedrol. The oil is steam-distilled from the *needles, twigs and cones.* It is anti-infectious and spasmolytic and a veinous decongestant. This Cypress is indicated for colitis or infections of the gut, to decongest the prostate and to stimulate pancreas and has primary use in the respiratory and circulatory systems. This is a warming, stimulating and uplifting oil and when inhaled just before bedtime can be soothing and relaxing. This Cypress is an astringent and helps to reduce overactive sweat and oil glands so can be used in bodycare for oily hair or skin or for sweaty palms or feet. As with many of the evergreen oils it is useful to reduce fluid retention and cellulite and for aching muscles, and arthritis pain. Emotional uses included smoothing transitions, especially when they involve the loss of loved ones or endings of relationships. It is inhaled for strength and comfort.

## **Group VI. Juniperus** (Junipers and other "Cedar"woods)

### ***Juniperus (Junipers).***

Trees of the *Juniperus genera* are the Junipers. Again, some of these essential oils are labled as Cedars, such as *Juniperus virginiana* which is sold as Virginia Cedar or "Cedarwood". Remember that True Cedars are of the Family *Pinaceae,* and are of the *Genera Cedrus,* yet *Juniperus virginiana* is obviously of the *Genera Juniperus* and of the family *Cupressaceæ* and it is still commonly called Virginia Cedar.

*Juniperus genera* plants have branchlets which are 4-angled, not in one plane. The fruit is a berry. The leaves are needle-shaped in whorls of 3.

Junipers include oil of "Cedarwood" from Virginia Cedar, *Juniperus virginiana,* contains mostly Cederene; oil of Texas

"Cedarwood" from *Juniperus mexicana*; oil of Juniper berries from *Juniperus communis*, used mainly in essences for flavoring beverages and liquers, particularly gin, used therapeutically as a diuretic; oil of *Juniperus oxycedrus*, the wood oil is called oil of Cade which is used in chronic excema; oil of Savin from *Juniperus sabina;* and others.

The essential oil from the wood of *J. virginiana* (often sold as "Cedar") is indicated for hemorrhoids and the wood is used for pencils or as a closet paneling. As was discussed in the Cedar section, many plants are called Cedarwood, but we are here discussing *Juniperus virginiana* which is used for the lining of closets to deter moths. Fragrant "Cedarwood" from *Juniperus virginiana* of the Cupressaceæ family, is used to line chests to repel vermin in the storage of valuables, especially furs and shoes. "Cedarwood" essential oil can be used in the same manner. Care should be taken that garments do not directly touch wood treated with "Cedarwood" essential oil.

Again, I will emphasize the importance of knowing that Latin binomial of the plant source of the essential oil you are using.

Now you can really see where the naming of these plants and essential oils becomes confusing with an oil called Cedar from the plant *Juniperus virginiana* with the common name Virginia Cedar. Again, this emphasizes the importance of informing yourself as to the Latin names of the essential oils, their sources, and their uses in comparison with the other essential oils in their family and genus. Very few retail essential oil companies provide this information on the label or in their price lists, so, at this point it is the responsibility of the consumer to inform themselves and to seek out responsible suppliers of essential oils.

*Juniperus communis* (common Juniper). Common Juniper is a native to the Northern Hemisphere. It is an evergreen shrub or tree up to 18 feet which has narrow, stiff, prickly needles and little brown berries that turn black in the second or third year. The essential oil is a steam distillation of the berries and has a very rich, deep aroma. Juniper berry essential oil contains 8% resins; 0.4% Juniperene; Pinene and Terpinenes. It is an expectorant and antiseptic and is used externally as a cleanser, and in massage oils and cosmetics. It has been used for urinary problems, genital warts, itchy vulva or jock

> I view aromatherapy as a branch of herbalism. Learning when use of the herb is preferable to use of the essential oil is an important aspect of aromatherapy training.

itch in the form of a sitz bath. Juniper berry essential oil can be taken in very small amounts to act as a diuretic for cystitis and to detoxify the body, but a tea of the berries is more highly recommended, especially mixed with Rosemary herb and Fennel seed. Juniper berries, 1 or 2, can be eaten as an aid to jet lag.

As with the other Evergreen oils, there are a variety of essential oils from a variety of Juniper plants, each with it's own indications.

The berry oil of subspecies *J. terpineoliferum* which is rich in Terpineols is used as a dissolver of kidney stones and used as a tonic for the digestive system and pancreas and is indicated for all sorts of treatments for the pancreas and kidney.

The essential oil from the wood of *J. mexicana* is used for hemorrhoids and to decongest the veinous system.

*Juniperus procera* (East African "Cedarwood"). Once again, although it is called a Cedar it is actually a Juniper.

In the case of *Juniperus oxycedrus* from the family *Cupressaceæ* the berry, leaf and wood are steam distilled to produce three different essential oils. The wood oil is generally called oil of Cade. It is an empyreumatic wood oil that is also commonly called oil of Juniper tar and often used in medicinal products for dandruff or scales on the skin such as might occur in eczema. It is also indicated for bad skin or greasy hair and is used in salves and ointments for minor skin irritations. It has been used to remove ticks from people and their pets by placing one drop of this oil on the skin close to the head of the tick. The tick can then be removed, counterclockwise. This plant is native to France and common in Europe and the tar is produced mainly in Spain and Yugoslavia. It is a large evergreen shrub, up to 12 feet. The Juniper tar is produced by destructive distillation of this particular Juniper. The process is called empyreumatic or partly decomposed. Components include a Sesquiterpene called Cadinene; Hydrocarbons and Phenols, among them Creosol. Cade fragrance is that of burning organic matter and combines well with Thyme, Oregano, or Clove.

*Juniperus sabina* (Savin). Mainly contains Sabinol and has *had* much use as an antirheumatic, vermifuge, and emmenogogue, but is *very* toxic and has had irritating side effects. The essential oil from the stems of *J. sabina* are used as an external application for rheumatism and occasionally to remove internal parasites.

You can see from the previous information that there are no hard and fast rules to giving common names to plants. Classifying and naming plant essential oils can also be a mess. Although many of the evergreen oils have similar uses, there are cases where it is important to know EXACTLY which oil you have or need. As with anything, the best way to clarify confusion is to do some research and experimentation. Especially, talk to the various essential oil distributors and retailers and get complete information about the oils you are purchasing, the Latin binomial, part of the plant used, country of origin. Buy a small quantity of the same oil from 2 disparate sources and compare color and scent. Remember that each year of growth, each harvest, each separate distillation will result in an oil with slightly different amounts of chemical components. The environment and individual ecology of a plant is important in the resultant essential oil. A year or two of great drought may result in a lower yield of essential oil but with improved or "stronger" components.

The fragrance of any particular essential oil varies from year to year and is totally dependent on the vagaries of "Mother Nature".

# Essential Oils of the Old Testament

Galbanum, Opopanax, and Cumin. Known to the centuries at least since 2000 BC and mentioned in the Old Testament, these are some of the herbs used in healing and as incense. But what do they have in common? Only that each contains an essential oil that is used in modern aromatherapy work.

Galbanum and Cumin are members of the Umbelliferae (now Apiaceae) family. Umbels are a cosmopolitan group of plants most often found in northern temperatures and tropical mountainous areas. They are herbs, that is, they usually do not develop persistent woody tissue, but they can also be shrubs and even trees. Umbels are usually aromatic and they are sometimes even poisonous *(Conium spp.)*. The flowers are usually small, bisexual and are united in compound umbels.

## Galbanum (*Ferula spp.* usually *F. galbaniflua*).

A large, perennial herb that is native to the Middle East. It looks like a large kind of Fennel. It is a strong rooted perennial with a flowering stem that reaches several feet in height. The leaves are finely divided and the umbels of flowers are greenish-white or yellow. The entire plant is rich in a milky juice which oozes from the joints of the plant, particularly older plants. This gum is an excretion which is gathered from the resinous ducts at the base of the shoots and leaves, and then hardens.

In the Old Testament, Galbanum grew on Mt. Amonus, in Syria. The name Galbanum comes from the Hebrew word *chalbaneh* which signifies something fat, unctuous and gummy. There are two types of Galbanum, one is soft and the other is hard. It was "an ingredient of the holy compound used in the Tabernacle (Ex. 30-34)." This holy scent was extremely important in Jewish observances. Maimonides, the Jewish philosopher who died in 1204 AD, says that the ancient incense was always *mixed* with salt from Sodom; but others think that Galbanum was *dissolved* in the salt and then used. Experts in incense-making were entrusted with the task of preparing the holy Galbanum incense and holy oil and in these ancient days it was forbidden for these plants to be used for any but a holy purpose. Whoever violated this law would "be swallowed up by the earth including all their families an all their goods" [1] However, in time, these peoples added the cleanly habits of the Egyptians—who practiced daily bathing—and so Galbanum came to be used not only as an incense and holy oil but in sweet ointments to be used after the bath. The Romans also imported the bathing habits of the Egyptians and refined the bath to include a system of sequential bathing—from hot tubs to warm to cold—and they too used all manner of sweet unctions including Galbanum. The Romans considered Galbanum to be the epitome of the color green and so it was used in ceremony when 'green' was to be invoked. Such is the ceremony of Spring to encourage the green growth of the new growing season.

Galbanum is soft (Levant) or hard (Persian). It can be dissolved in alcohol yielding a yellow tincture. Chemical composition shows the following: d-α-Pinene up to 12%, β-Pinene up to 45%, Myrcene, an unknown component which possesses the typical 'green' or Bell Pepper odor of Galbanum and which has the formula $C_{10}H_{16}0$, Cadinene and a-Cadinol. The oil is obtained by S-D from the gum.

Galbanum oil is considered a tonic stimulant that is anti-infectious and is used by inhalation to resolve old problems, particularly old problems of an emotional nature. It is indicated for all types of menstrual problems and women's care, particularly by application in a massage blend, to apply to the skin to heal old skin lesions and as a tool for meditation. In previous years it was used as a stimulating inhalant, antispasmodic and expectorant. The scent of Galbanum oil is warm, earthy and green. It is very specific, once you have smelled it you will never forget it. You will either like it or dislike it. The scent is truly indescribable. Two to three drops in an 8-oz blend of essential oils is enough to 'fix' the scent and add a deep quality to the blend that is both uplifting, very grounding and earthy.

### Cumin *(Cuminum cyminum).*

Cumin is also called Cummin in older texts. It is a small, slender annual herb with finely dissected leaves, white or pinkish flowers

[1] Rimmel, Eugene. *The Book of Perfumes.* London: Chapman and Hall, 1865.

and a fruit that looks like a miniature ball with bristles. Cumin is native, from the Meditteranean area to the Sudan. It has been cultivated here since the times of the Minoans, about 1300 BC. It is also cultivated in India, where it forms part of the mixture called Curry Powder, and in China and Mexico as well. Cumin is mentioned in both the Old and New Testament; in Matthew 23:23, it is discussed as a plant that could be used to pay the tax, "For Ye pay tithe of Mint and Anise and Cumin."

To use the Cumin seed, harvest the umbels when the seeds within are ripe, brownish in color, and spread them in a warm, dry, airy place. When the Umbels and seeds are thoroughly dry, shake the Umbels gently so that the seeds fall out on paper that you have laid down to catch them. Store the seeds in a paper bag in a dry, dark place. The seeds are crushed and then steam-distilled for up to 12 hours to produce the essential oil which has a peculiar scent; warm, strong and very reminiscent of the scent of curried foods. The seeds produce about 2.5% essential oil and it is advised that the distillation water is redistilled to extract all the essential oil—that is, cohobate the distillation water. Seeds from different areas produce varying yields of oil, from up to 5% from Malta seeds to 2.3 to 3.5% from East Indian seeds. The chemical composition includes d-l-Pinene and d-α-Pinene, p-Cymene, β-Pinene, Dipentene, Cuminaldehyde which constitutes 35-62% of the total, Dihydrocuminaldehyde is present in small quantities and Cuminyl Alcohol. Often the oil is adulterated with synthetic Cuminaldehyde and this usually cannot be

**Compounds exist in the following percentages**

|  |  |
|---|---|
| α - Pinene | 1.3 to 2.6 |
| Camphene | 2.4 to 9.0 |
| δ - Pinene | 4.5 to 15.0 |
| Limonene | 6.0 to 16.0 |
| p - Cymene | 10.3 to 14.3 |
| Cuminaldehyde | 21.9 to 28.5 |
| Cuminyl ester | 25.1 to 31.6 |

detected except by examining the optical rotation of the oil molecule.

Cumin oil is considered calming to the nerves when inhaled, to the point of stupefication, it is a strong antispasmodic to the digestive system and stimulates digestion when taken internally. In this case it can be added to foods to produce a strong Indian or Mexican flavour to the food, 1 drop per serving for medicinal use and 1 drop per four servings as flavor. Cumin oil is indicated as a tonic for dyspepsia and gas and spasms in the gut, it can be inhaled for insomnia, taken for low thyroid function and used as a treatment externally as well as internally for orchitis. In 1988, a study using Cumin oil showed that an aqueous extract of Cumin seeds possessed antifertility and abortifacient activity when administered to female rats.[2]

## Opopanax (Bisabol-Myrrh).

Another ancient plant is Opopanax. It is a member of the Burseraceæ family which also includes Linaloe, Myrrh, Olibanum (Frankincense) and Elemi. These plants are closely related to the Umbels. Guenther states that in the past "true Opopanax meant the concrète juice or oleo-gum-resin of *Opopanax chironium* which is related to the Parsnip and is native to the warm countries of the Levant"[3]. But apparently this type is no longer available and what is found on the market is a Bisabol-Myrrh, the sun-dried exudation from the bark of *Commiphora erythraea* which is a tall tree growing in the western part of Somaliland. The ancient Opopanax was used as an antispasmodic while modern Opopanax is generally considered an anti-inflammatory useful to the practitioner as a deterrent to internal parasites.

Opopanax contains Bisabolene and other components including resins and gums. The compounds that are chiefly responsible for the strong and interesting odor have not yet been identified. Guenther describes the odor as interesting while I feel that it seems a cross between Olibanum and Myrrh with an elusive 'bite'.

Bisabol-Myrrh is a valuable ingredient in perfumery because of its warm, balsamic, and exotic odor. It works well in perfumes and

[2] Brian M. Lawrence. Monographs on Essential Oils. *Perfumer and Flavourist.* Carol Sream: Allured Publishing, 1975-94.

[3] Guenther, Ernest. *The Essential Oils.* Malabar, FL: Krieger Publishing Co., 1976.

blends that have an oriental character and as a fixative. The animal-sweet nature of the scent works well in inhalation therapy to 'free one from evil thoughts' and as an aid in meditation. This oil is indicated for use in blends to heal skin ulcers. For skin-care, see *The Herbal Body Book* by Jeanne Rose, Opopanax (all-healing vegetable juice) has many uses.

Remember when reading about Opopanax/Bisabol-Myrrh that there is much confusion regarding terminology and it is best to rely on the Latin name rather than the common name when deciding how to use the essential oil.

These are just three of the Old Testament plants that yield an essential oil.

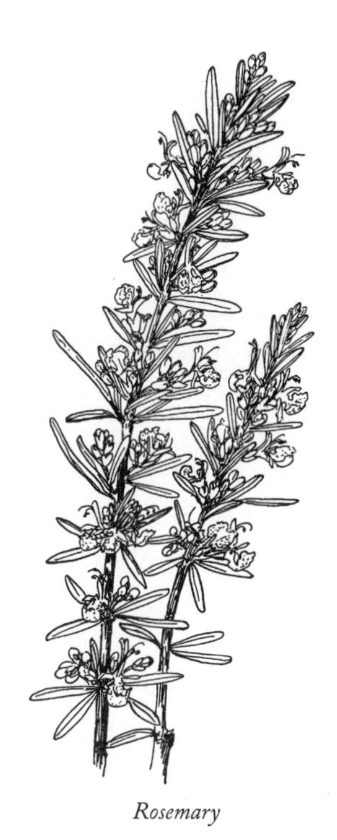

*Rosemary*

## The Roots of Aroma

Many species of plants whose foliage and flowers may not be particularly fragrant are quite at home in the aromatic garden because of their aromatic roots.

***Asarum,*** commonly known as **Ginger** or **Wild Ginger,** the most pungently scented species are native to Canada and California. These plants are perennial herbs with a creeping rootstock and long-stalked, heart-shaped leaves. *Asarum* grows best in humus-laden, well-watered soil and are considered a delicacy by slugs and snails.

*A. canadense,* (Canadian snakeroot), produces brownish-purple flowers in early summer that are so unpleasant it is hard to believe that any part of the plant has a pleasant smell. When dried, the roots have a strong ginger odor.

*A. canadatum,* a native to California and also produces reddish-brown, unpleasantly scented flowers. It blooms earlier and has a less aromatic root than *A. canadense,* although the root does smell of ginger.

***Zingiber,*** **True Ginger,** of the *Zingiber* genus has a strong, spicy aroma. The rhizomes and roots are steam-distilled for an essential oil that is used in the perfume trade to give "warmth" to a blend. One drop of Ginger essential oil in Ginger Ale or carbonated water is drunk before dining as an aperitif or to ease gas or stomach pains after eating. Compresses or baths including Ginger essential oil can be used to reduce fever or pain. Externally the essential oil is used for muscular aches and pains, for arthritis, rheumatism, chest pains from cold or flu, or sore throat or swollen glands. In this regard it can be used as a compress or in a massage oil. It is a stimulant and when mixed with Rosemary can be used as a wake-up inhalation. It eases mental confusion and is said to "warm the heart." As a stimulating, warming oil it is well used by the traveler.

***Inula helenium*** **(Elecampane)** was botanically named Inula because its roots yield a starch called inulin, from which certain sugars are obtained.

The species *helenium* was named in honor of Helen of Troy. Elecampane, the largest of all British wildflowers, is steeped in history. It is a tall and regal herb, with oversized, pointed leaves covered in fine hair. It generally grows to four or five feet, but if planted in a shady spot in rich soil, may grow to more than ten feet. The flowers are yellow to orange, daisy-like, fringed, and have been compared to miniature double sunflowers.

Elecampane harbors its strong scent in its roots, which at first smell like ripe bananas then like violets as they age. At one time the roots were eaten as vegetables or candied as sweetmeat. The powdered root has been praised in the treatment of bronchial ailments.

***Vetiveria zizanioides*** **Vetiver** in America, was one of the most popular scents for men's cologne during the 1950s and 1960s. In India, *V. zizanioides* formed the base of a substance called mousseline, named for Indian muslin that had been doused in its perfume.

*V. zizanioides* has swordlike, tapering leaves with strong, rooty, violet-scented, rhizomatous roots. The best way to have the plants for garden growth is to plant them in plastic containers which can be sunk into the garden and covered with mulch. *V. zizanioides* grows in moderate light with average soil, and will also thrive in poor soil and full sun. Once a year the pots should be lifted, plants removed, roots trimmed, then the plants re-potted and replaced in the garden.

Fragrant baskets and sunblinds can be made from the abundant, dense, fibrous mats produced by roots of the adult plants. The roots are easily dried and give a distinct scent to potpourri.

The essential oil of Vetiver (also known as Vetivert or Khus-Khus) is S-D from the roots to produce a thick, green essential oil. The scent is clean, refreshing, and slightly woody. It is used in perfumery and potpourris as a fixative, and in lotions to stimulate circulation for aching joints. It is moisturizing, so is also useful for dry, irritated, mature, or aging skin. It blends well with other oils for this purpose, such as Rose, Frankincense, Myrrh, and Patchouli. Vetiver is the oil of choice used in place of Sandalwood, which is now becoming extinct from over-cultivation. The aroma of Vetiver is grounding, calming, and sedating and affects the parathyroid glands.

# Essential Oil Profiles

## *Ammi visnaga* (Ammi visnaga)

*Common Name:* Ammi
*Family:* Apiaceae
*Most important use:* Allergic asthma
*Purchasing Guide:* The color is deep golden yellow to warm golden brown. The deeper the color the more viscous (or thick) the oil. The odor is rich, deep, aromatic, and very memorable. The more you inhale the odor, the more it can be upsetting to your stomach.
*Availability:* Best places to obtain are mail order: Prima Fleur (415-455-0957), and Original Swiss Aromatics (415-479-9120)
*Countries of Origin:* Mediterranean, North Africa, Morocco
*Other Common Names:* Toothpick plant, Spanish carrot, carotte cure-dent, herbe aux cure-dents, swak en-nebi, khelal, khellin
*History:* A tea made from the seeds of this plant has been in use for centuries as an anti-asthmatic and for other respiratory problems. In 1897, a major constituent was isolated in crystalline form and called "khellin". This was found on examination to be a relaxant on various types of smooth muscle tissue, i.e., the gut and bronchial tubes. However, the point at which the tea eases an asthmatic attack is also where it causes nausea and vomiting. The oil was studied in India and the noxious element was chemically removed. Ultimately this compound came to be called cromolyn sodium and is used in modern respiratory medicine. When cromolyn sodium is inhaled, it masks the function of the mast cells thereby decreasing attacks of allergic asthma. *Ammi visnaga* can also be used as an inhalant with other essential oils such as *Rosemary pyramidalis* and *Eucalyptus smithii.* The seed is often used in tincture form with other herbs such as turmeric, which acts as an anti-inflammatory. However, too much of the tincture can also result in nausea and vomiting. (Take only 10 drops 3x/day.)
*Description of plant:* The plant is very similar in appearance to the Carrot or Umbelliferae family. It is an annual plant growing up to two feet high, with a longish white root. The stem is erect, fluted

and round. The plant branches at the top with delicate leaves repeatedly divided. The leaves become thin wisps just like the carrot. The umbel arises from a branching base, often with more than 100 rays or stalks 4-5 cm in length, each with a small umbel of numerous white flowers eventually with small egg-shaped elliptical fruits that are smooth, grayish brown. The leaves have a bitter taste and aromatic scent. "To 2.5 feet; leaves finely divided into linear threadlike segments; umbels spreading in flowers, 60-100 rays borne on a disc, to 4 inches long, as long as the divided involucral bracts, fruits to 3/32 in. long. Southern Europe naturalized in North America. Cultivated for its potential as a drug." (*Hortus Third)*

*Part Used:* Fresh and dried seeds are used as a tea and the seeds are steam distilled to yield the oil. Components are monoterpenes, esters, and chromones, mainly 1% khelline.

*Properties and Uses:* Seeds are diuretic, appetizer, carminative, stimulant, emmenogogue, lithontriptic (able to dissolve or release stones from bladder or kidney), and useful for all types of urinary disorders, angina, asthma, or gastric ulcers. An infusion of the seeds is used in all these cases. The essential oil is inhaled or can be taken internally and used as an antispasmodic, coronary dilator, bronchodilator, and anticoagulant. A doctor's recommendation is valuable for internal uses of this oil. The essential oil is indicated for insufficiency of the heart muscle, atherosclerosis, asthma, colitis, and liver disturbance.

*Interesting information:* For prophylactic use, an inhalant of *Ammi visnaga* (or cromolyn sodium, Intal®) is used to mask the function of the mast cells to relieve symptoms of allergic asthma. There is much coumarin and cromone in the Mediterranean plant, but these components are detected only in traces in plants grown in the United States.

*Contraindications:* Can cause photosensitization when used externally.

## ***Cedrus atlantica*** or ***C. deodora***

*Common Name:* Cedar or True Cedar

*Family:* Pinaceae

*Most important use:* Oily skin and hair

*Purchasing Guide:* I purchased samples from six different companies.

| *Cedrus atlantica* | A | B | C | D | E | F |
|---|---|---|---|---|---|---|
| taste | exotic wood and fruit | | | | | |
| color | 24k | 24k | 22k | 22k | 20k | 20k |
| scent | rich depth | airy & woods | deep woods | rich depth | balsam resin | resin & wood |
| cost/ml | .214 | .30 | unknown | .46 | unknown | .29 |

I am happy to report that I could rate *Cedrus atlantica* color according to the color of the metal gold. All were lovely and tinted deep gold; all of the samples had the same deep levels of scent, woody, fruity overtones with deep balancing energy; the taste of all the samples was as identical as the scent, like biting into a piece of deeply fragrant wood with a bit of a bite, the taste also made my mouth water and was actually quite pleasant with an exotic tropical fruitiness.

Since all of these samples were superior in color, scent and taste and the only difference was price, my suggestion is that you buy this product from the nearest company listed here. This is a wonderful oil to learn and use.

*Availability:* A is Prima Fleur at 415/455-0957
B is Original Swiss Aromatics at 415/479-9120
C is a distributor, Fleurom at 336/282-9734
D is Phytosun Aromatherapy
E is an unknown sample
F is Oshadhi

*Countries of Origin: Cedrus atlantica* Manetti (fam. Pinaceae) occurs in the Atlas Mountains of Morocco and Algeria.

*History:* There are several very different woods that are called Cedarwood. The most usual ones named are: *Juniperus virginiana,* red Cedarwood from the Native American tree of the family Cupressaceae; Oil of Cade which results from the destructive distillation of the wood of *Juniperus oxycedrus* (fam. Cupressaceae), Oil of Thuja plicata which contains a highly poisonous ketone and is obtained from the heartwood of the Western Red Cedar, *Thuja plicata* (fam. Cupressaceae) and the true Cedarwood oil which is obtained from *Cedrus atlantica* or *C. deodora* (fam. Pinaceae).

It is obvious when reading aromatherapy books and magazines that many authors do not realize how confusing it is when only common names for the essential oils are used. It is to be hoped that in the future these same authors will begin to list the essential oils not only by common name but by Latin binomial as well. In an Autumn issue of a popular newsletter, two popular books were reviewed in which the Virginia 'Cedar' was listed as the timber used in the building of the temple of Solomon. Clearly, this is incorrect as the Virginia 'Cedar" is a Newe Worlde plant and was not named until it was found and identified in North America in the 1500's.

*Description of Plant: Cedrus atlantica Manetti* (fam. Pinaceae), the so-called "Atlas Cedar," is a tall tree attaining a height of about 40 m.

*Parts Used:* Wood is distilled for the EO.

*Properties and Uses:* Guenther lists the composition as Sesquiterpenes, δ-Cadinene, and γ-Atlantone which is the chief constituent of the oil.

Oil of Atlas Cedarwood is used both in its local habitat and elsewhere in the world against all kinds of respiratory disease as an inhalant or externally as an application for skin disease. In natural perfume blending, and blending of essential oil formulas, this oil is an excellent odor fixative and 'loses itself' when mixed with other essential oils. Other properties are as an arterial regenerative and lymphotonic. It aids in the removal of body fat, and is used externally for cellulite and edema (fluid retention) in the body. Atlas Cedar is a good oil for the medicine chest; a drop in a half cup of water is gargled for sore throat or with a few drops of Eucalyptus in a bowl of steaming water and inhaled reduces nasal and lung congestion.

Atlas Cedarwood oil can also be used in the body care industry; added to shampoos or facial washes to reduce oily secretions. *Cedrus atlantica* is non toxic orally, when used neat is a very mild skin irritant, does not cause sensitization and is not photo-toxic according to Essential Oil Safety.

*Interesting Information:* According to some authorities this tree is closely related to the Lebanon Cedar. This famous tree, *Cedrus libani* is possibly the oldest perfume material known. The trees are protected on Cyprus and in Lebanon and the essential oil is no longer used.

*Contraindications:* None known.

## ***Pelargonium graveolens*** or ***P. asperum*** Pelargonium oil, Rose Geranium oil, or Geranium oil

*Family:* Geraniaceae

*Most important use:* Skin care. Conditions relating to women's reproductive organs

*Purchasing Guide:* The color of this oil ranges from a deep golden yellow to yellow to clear emerald green. The emerald green oil comes from plantings that have been made in California in the United States from *P. graveolens,* while the oil simply labeled Geranium is golden-yellow-brown from China. Geranium Bourbon from Morocco and Madagascar is pale yellowish-green. Cost: $8-9 per ½ oz. wholesale, up to $30 per ½ oz. retail. It pays to shop around for the best quality at the best price.

The scent of the oil is eponymous—an herby green odor with rose-like overtones and a deep rich undertone of mint and citrus.

*Availability:* This essential oil is easily obtainable from a variety of sources, and ranges from standardized oils for commercial skin care products to exquisite selections used mainly for therapeutic aroma uses.

*Countries of Origin:* Morocco, Madagascar, Egypt, China and California. Unfortunately, though the plant is indigenous to South Africa, at this time this lovely product is not available from this country.

*Other Common Names:* None.

Popularly known as scented geraniums, these plants are actually scented Pelargonium. Unlike the common garden geraniums, they belong to the genus *Pelargonium.* The generic name, from the Greek *pelargos,* "stork", comes from the notion that the long, narrow seed capsule resembled a stork's bill. Storksbill is also an old common name. The word *graveolens* means 'heavily scented'. Pelargoniums belong to the geranium family (Geraniaceae), as does the genus *Geranium,* which includes cranesbills and herb Robert.

The taxonomy of the plants cultivated in various areas of the world is a matter of controversy and confusion. Geranium, the name itself, is a misnomer as Geranium oil comes from the true Geranium plant, a common garden plant, *Geranium macrorrhizum L.* This plant grows wild in Bulgaria and other Balkan countries and is used for the distillation of an oil called Zdravetz (meaning health).

On the other hand, true Pelargonium oil comes from *P. graveolens* or *P. asperum* or a cross of these two. Pelargonium plants readily cross and they change their oil components, quality, and quantity, depending on where grown. Rose geranium (*Pelargonium*) oil *does not* come from the garden plants called *P. odoratissimum*, which is a small trailing plant whose leaves have the odor of nutmeg or green apples, nor does it come from the garden plant called *P. fragrans*, which is also not suitable for cultivation.

*History and Growing Conditions:* The great part of the world's supply of Pelargonium oil comes from the island of Reunion (Bourbon), a very fertile island about 400 miles east of Madagascar. The plant was introduced to the island in about 1880. The original plant grown for essential oil production was different from that cultivated today. In about 1900 *P. graveolens* was introduced from Grasse in France and was a plant that grew larger and more bushy, and therefore produced more oil—and the oil was of a sweeter, more rose-like odor. Since Pelargoniums change and develop according to the climate and soil type in which they are grown, the essential oil of Reunion also changed and altered. Reunion oil contains more citronellol than that grown in France and less than that grown in Egypt and China. Pelargonium plants like a soil that is neither moist nor dry, a temperate climate with sea moisture (such as occurs in San Francisco) and do not like periods of heavy rain or torrid heat.

Cuttings of this plant have been taken throughout the world and various plantings have been started.

*Description of the Plant:* A perennial hairy shrub up to 3-4 feet in height. It is shrubby, erect, branching, hairy, densely leafy; the leaves are triangular, cordate at the base, deeply five-lobed, hairy, grey-green, rose-scented; peduncle, 5-10 flowered; petals, small, pink; upper veined and spotted purple. *P. asperum* is often considered to be unpleasantly scented with few flowers of pale lilac.

The scent is contained in small beads of oil produced in glands at the base of tiny leaf hairs. Bruising or crushing a leaf breaks the beads and releases their fragrance.

Pelargonium thrives in light porous soil which is friable and does not retain moisture. It is easily propagated by cuttings. The essential oil is contained in small glands that are distributed over the green parts of the plant, particularly over the surface of the leaves. The glands can be seen by the naked eye and give to the leaf its silvery satin-like sheen. The yield of oil is higher when the plant is allowed to wither for a few hours prior to distillation. However, for the greatest amount of hydrosol, the plant is steam-distilled as soon as possible after it is picked.

*Part Used:* The top third of the plant is cut, up to four times per year, and is steam-distilled to yield the oil and hydrosol. Generally, the heavier stalks are removed prior to distillation. The wood absolutely must be excluded from the distillation process. The yield of oil varies from ½ kg per 250 kg of freshly picked material. The amount is higher in the summer cut than the winter (just after winter) cut. In California where we mostly try to get great quality hydrosol, 200 lbs of leaf material cut and distilled in August, produced 1 ounce of emerald green essential oil and 50 gallons of hydrosol.

*Physiochemical Properties—According to Gunther.* The Réunion geranium oil possesses a very strong, heavy rose-like odor, occasionally slightly harsh and minty. The oil is valued particularly on acccount of its high citronellol content, which makes the Réunion type of geranium oil the best starting material for the extraction of commercial "rhodinol."

*Properties and Uses:* Skin care: Used externally on acne, bruises, as a tonic astringent application for broken capillaries, burns, couperose skin, cuts, all types of skin conditions, externally for hemorrhoids, in products for oily or mature skin. Used externally in massage for cellulite, breast engorgement, edema, or poor circulation. Used by inhalation for menopausal symptoms or PMS, ner-

**Comparison of Main Components**

| Compound | California | Bourbon | Egyptian | Chinese |
|---|---|---|---|---|
| citronellyl formate | 21.78% | | | |
| citronellol | 34.82% | 22-40% | 30-38% | 45-51% |
| geraniol | 6.86% | 14-18% | 16-17% | 5-7% |

vous tension, or stress. Used extensively in the skin-care industry for all types of cosmetic problems. The hydrosol is excellent as a spray tonic for the skin, to reduce stress, relieve all sorts of menstrual or menopausal symptoms. As an inhalant the EO is considered to balance the adrenocortical glands. Used internally by ingestion for the liver and pancreas (with the assistance of a health care provider). This oil is considered to be anti-infectious, anti-bacterial, anti-fungal (Spikenard is better), anti-inflammatory, relaxing, and anti-spasmodic.

*Interesting Information:* This plant produces quite different oils depending on the environment, climate, soil, elevation. Take several cuttings of a mother plant and plant each cutting in different parts of the world; within three years, depending on the environmental and ecological conditions you will have as many different oils with varying components as you have different environments.

*Contraindications:* None known.

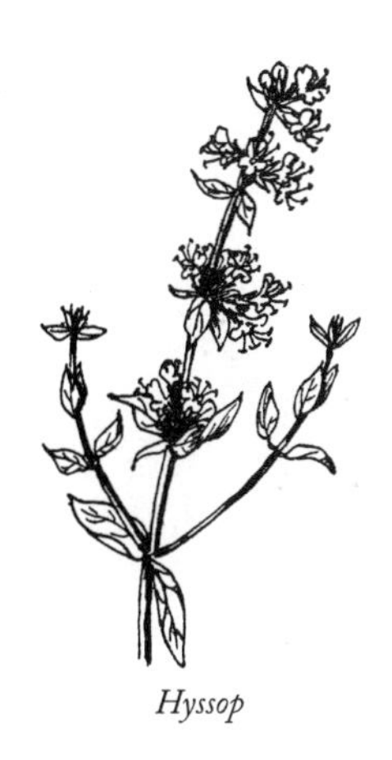
*Hyssop*

# EIGHT

# How To Use Essential Oils and Hydrosols

Essential Oils and Hydrosols can be applied in three basic ways: application, inhalation, and internal; furthermore, internal use can be culinary (in or on foods), by ingestion in capsules or on charcoal or throat lozenges, and via suppositories that can be used in the rectum, vagina, ear canal or urethra, any bodily opening.

Application of essential oils and hydrosols can be applied via massage, a bath, a compress, or through body care products. Essential oils are used in a 2% solution, that is, 2 drops of EO to every 98 drops of carrier substance. With hydrosols, you can spritz them just about anywhere. Some ideas for use are given at the end of this chapter.

Essential oils can be inhaled straight from the bottle, from a diffuser or nebulizer, or from a hanky or pillowcase that has been spritzed. Essential oils can also be inhaled through vaporization in a bowl of hot water: use only 1–2 drops at a time. Hydrosols can be used as a nasal wash or sprayed into any other orifice to clear it.

Internal use of essential oils and hydrosols is still somewhat controversial here in the United States. It is best to remember that no more than 100 mg. (about 4 drops) of an essential oil is suggested to be taken on any one day, particularly if you are a beginner in the uses of EO. (1 drop = about 25 mg. and 30 drops = about 1 ml.) So remember when reading formulas to respect the difference between milliliters (ml.) and milligrams (mg.). I personally make an essential oil formula and then add drops to a capsule that also affects the condition I am treating. For instance, to treat my asthma, I use base capsules of *Ginkgo biloba,* take one apart, add the required amount of essential oils, put the capsule back together, and swallow it with water.

Hydrosols can be added to water. Place 3–4 tablespoons in a liter of water, and then drink that water throughout the day. Rose Geranium hydrosol water is particularly good for women with any sort of menstrual problems or who are going through menopause. Lavender and Lavandin hydrosol is effective for calming children or calming distress in general. Lemon verbena hydrosol water can be drunk for a virus infection or sprayed when the infection is external. Lemon balm hydrosol water can be drunk throughout the day to focus attention; it is particularly good for students and can be used as well for viral infections.

Suppositories made with essential oils are an effective way to treat digestive and respiratory problems. To make suppositories: Find your smallest pot or double boiler. Melt 2 tablespoons of cocoa butter (a 1 x 1 x 1 inch cube or 20 g. ) with 1 dr. (1/8 oz. or 3 ½ ml.) of hazelnut or olive oil. Be careful so that you do not burn or heat up these fats too much—you only want to melt them. To help prevent overheating or burning, you can use a small bowl placed in a pot of hot water and heat gently. When the fats are melted, remove the pot from the burner or the bowl from the water to a table and add 1 dr. (105–120 drops or 3 ½ ml.) of your mixture of essential oils.

Incorporate the two ingredients, and let it cool. Then pour or spoon the mixture into a folded piece of aluminum foil. The aluminum foil should be 4 inches wide, about a foot long. Fold in the ends along the long side and fold in half the long way so that you have a trough about 10 inches long. Spread the mixture along the fold, and roll the foil so that you create a long, round, pencil-shaped roll of suppository.* Freeze. After it is frozen, cut into 15 pieces. Each of these suppositories (pieces) will contain about 6 drops of the essential oil mixture. Use no more than 2 per day (adults only, not for children) and for no more than 5 days, unless recommended by a trained aromamedicalist.

---

*Suppositories are used in any opening of the body; vagina, rectum, ears, or urethra.

These are very general instructions for the use of essential oils and hydrosols. *The Aromatherapy Book: Applications & Inhalations* has more specific instructions.

**Measurement Chart in Drops, Milligrams, milliliters**

| | |
|---|---|
| 1 oz. = | 29.75 ml |
| 1 ml. = | 29–30 measured drops (depending on the size of the dropper opening) |
| 1 drop = | 15 mg. (Penoël) or 25 mg. (Schnaubelt) |
| 150 mg. = | 10 drops (Penoël) or 6 drops (Schnaubelt) |

(The difference in amounts between Penoël and Schnaubelt are due to the different sizes of the openings of droppers.)

Remember that milliliters (ml.) is a volume measurement while milligrams (mg.) is a weight measurement. Since not many of us have a milligram scale, it is often easier to use milliliter as a measurement. (A measured milliliter dropper can be obtained from any pharmacy.) Ounces (oz.) can be either volume or weight and are not a reliable indicator of precise essential oil measurements.

## How to Use Essential Oils and Hydrosols

**Bath Water** Add 5–15 drops of EO to tub of warm water. Swish with hand to mix. The number of drops used depends on the size of the bath tub. Use the larger amount for a deeper bath.

**Body Lotion or Oil** Use 1/2–1 teaspoon EO per pint of unscented body lotion or botanical oil such as sunflower or Olive or other oil or 2 drops to 1 dram.

**Candles** Light candle and wait for wax to begin melting. Add 1–2 drops of EO to melting wax, being careful not to get flammable oil on burning wick.

**Carpet Freshener** Mix 1 teaspoon EO with 1/2 cup each baking soda and cornstarch. Blend well with mortar and pestle or spoon. Set for 30 minutes. Sprinkle on carpet, wait 30 minutes, then vacuum. If you substitute Borax for the soda and starch, and leave it on the carpet overnight, you can also kill the fleas and mites.

**Cotton Balls** Put 1–3 drops on cotton ball to diffuse scent. Put the cotton balls in your drawers, in bed clothes or clothes closet. Lavender oil promotes restful sleep.

**Measurement Chart Conversion Table***

*Liquids:*

| Apothecary Doses | Metric System Doses |
|---|---|
| 1 quart | 1000 cc. [a cubic centimeter (cc.) is 1/1000 of a liter] |
| 1 pint | 500 cc. |
| 8 fluid ounces | 240 cc. |
| 3 ½ fluid ounces | 100 cc. |
| 1 fluid ounce | 30 cc. |
| 4 fluid drams | 15 cc. |
| 1 fluid dram | 4 cc. |
| 15 minims (drops) | 1 cc. |
| 1 minim (drop) | 0.06 cc. |

*Solids:*

| Apothecary Doses | Metric System Doses |
|---|---|
| 1 ounce | 30 grams |
| 4 drams | 15 grams |
| 1 dram | 4 grams |
| 60 grains (1 dram) | 4 grams |
| 30 grains (½ dram) | 2 grams |
| 15 grains | 1 gram |
| 10 grains | 0.6 grams |
| 1 grain | 60 milligram (mg.) |
| ¾ grain | 50 mg. |
| ½ grain | 30 mg. |
| ¼ grain | 15 mg. |
| 1/6 grain | 10 mg. |
| 1/10 grain | 6 mg. |
| 1/100 grain | 0.6 mg |

**all equivalents are approximate*

**Culinary** 1 drop EO per 4 servings in salad dressings, sauces, desserts, or beverages.

**Diffusers** These special products include the lamp ring diffuser, car diffuser, tabletop diffuser, glass mister, and room diffuser. Diffusers work with as little as 10 drops of oil. At highest setting 1 dram in 2 hours or at lowest setting 1 dram in 12 hours.

**Drawer & Shelf Liners** Put several drops on cotton and wipe down liners or just add several drops directly to the liner. Avoid contact with clothing or linen until oil is dry, as some oils stain fabrics. Bay, Basil, Pine, and Fir are good oils for kitchen cupboards.

**Facial Waters** Add 6–8 drops per ounce of pure water and spritz on the face. Lavender, Rose, and Orange EO make wonderful facial waters.

**Herbal Sachets** Add several drops of EO to moth-repelling dry herbs (e.g., Cedar and Sage) in muslin bags. Choose oil(s) compatible with the dry herb(s) used.

**House Cleaning Water** In a quart of water, put 4–8 drops EO and 3–4 tablespoons white vinegar to improve cleaning action. Use on counter tops, in cabinets, and in mop water. Eucalyptus, Lemon, Lavandin, Peppermint, Rose Geranium, Rosemary, and Thyme are good choices to scent, clean, and disinfect.

**Humidifier** Add 6–8 drops to water in humidifier.

**Hydrosols** These are a product of distillation and can be added to any liquid or lotion in a ratio of 1 part hydrosol to 3 parts other. Use undiluted as a refreshing and healing spritz. Spritz for hot flashes, or to cool the skin. Use after cleansing the face as a toner, and after applying make-up to set it. Spritz for diaper rash. Use in the last rinse of hand-washables for pleasant aroma. Spritz hot spots on animals for healing. Use as aftershave spritz to tone and soothe the skin.

**Laundry Rinse** Add 2–3 drops EO per quart of water. Use this dilution for hand washables or add to washing-machine cup for final rinse. You can also add water to your empty essential oil bottles and pour into final rinse or in the fabric softener container in your machine.

**Light Bulbs** Put several drops or Lemon Eucalyptus or Citronella oil on cool outdoor lights before illuminating to repel insects.

Make sure EO does not drip into the socket. Indoors, use a lamp ring diffuser to efficiently release scents when lights are turned on.

**Massage** 5–15 drops EO per ounce of base oil for massage (amount depends on EO used).

**Perfumery** Most essential oils are too concentrated to apply to skin undiluted. To make your own perfume, blend 1 dram EO with 3 drams ethyl alcohol. For milder fragrance, make your eau de toilette with 15 drops EO, 50 drops ethyl alcohol or 60% vodka, and 30–40 drops distilled water. Age 2 weeks before using. Shake well before each use.

**Pet Grooming** After bath, use 2 drops Rosemary, Rose Geranium, or Lavandin in a pint of water as a conditioning rinse for pets. Between shampoos, soak pet's brush in 2 drops of Lavender, Tea Tree or Cedarwood Oil per pint warm water. Shake out excess and use to brush coat with conditioning, flea-repelling scents.

**Potpourri** Revive the faded bloom on potpourri with a few drops of EO. Stir to disperse scents. Cover for 2 weeks before use.

**Room Spray** 4 drops per cup of warm (not hot) water. Use a new plant mister to diffuse into the air. Avoid contact with wood furniture.

**Scented Books & Paper** Use a few drops of repellent oils (Clove, Lavender, or Rosemary) on absorbent papers to make scented bookmarks that also repel bugs. Scent stationery with a little oil to make your letters fragrantly memorable. (Do not use on old, treasured books.)

**Water-Bowl Room Freshener** 1–9 drops oil in a small bowl of warm water scents a room. Put water bowl on radiator, allowing heat to release the scents.

**Wood Fires** Put 1 drop on each log ½ hour *before* starting fire.

## Hydrosols

As a product of distillation, hydrosols can be added to any liquid or lotion in a ratio of 1 part hydrosol to 3 parts other material. Hydrosols can also be used undiluted as a refreshing and healing spritz. They can be used in all the ways that are mentioned above.

**Baby** Spritz to soothe diaper rash.

**Face** Spritz with hydrosol for hot flashes and/or to cool the skin. Use as a toner after cleansing the face or use to set makeup.

**Laundry** Spritz in the last rinse of hand washables for pleasant aroma.

**Pets** Spritz sensitive areas on animals for healing and soothing.

**Shaving** Use as aftershave spritz to tone and soothe the skin.

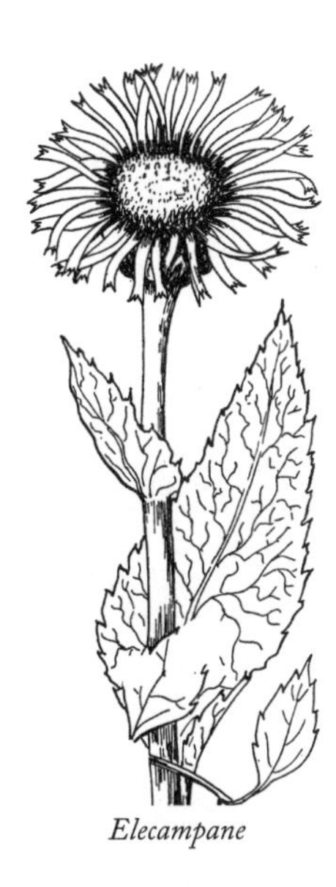

*Elecampane*

# NINE

# Sources 2000

Over the years, I have published various source lists for the consumer. These source lists were given to aid the consumer and enable them to know where to go and where to purchase quality herbal and aromatic products. Please note, that phone numbers change it seems weekly, locations change as a business grows, and sometimes websites are hard to find. So addresses only are given. For quality products, *write* a postcard to the following addresses. Request a product and/or a price list. Get several product and/or price lists and purchase an oil or hydrosol from each source. Compare both for price, quality, and service. See what sort of response you get from your request postcard. Than choose a company that you wish to give your business to.

Currently, these are my favorite source companies:

Australian Essential Oil Company. 575 Myall Creek Road. P.O. Box 158. Coraki 2471. NSW. Australia. Has developed the fabulous Blue Cypress and other oils from indigenous plants.

The Aromatic Plant Project. 219 Carl Street. San Francisco, CA 94117. Aromatherapy education with a Certificate Course and the developer of locally-grown, perfectly-distilled hydrosols for your every day needs. This non-profit organization supports American agriculture. Phone (415) 564-6785.

CH Imports. P.O. Box 18411. Greensboro, NC. 27419. Wholesale and retail essential oils and aromatherapy ingredients. Carries a wonderful Hydrosol still for home use.

Essential Aromatics. 205 N. Signal Street. Ojai, CA 93023. A wonderful retail product line with a variety of products and essential oil and aromatherapy candles.

Essentially Oils, Ltd. 8 Mount Farm. Junction Road, Churchill. Chipping Norton. Oxfordshire. OX7 6NP. United Kingdom. Always an interesting and unique listing of wonderful quality essential oils.

Jeanne Rose Aromatherapy. 219 Carl Street. San Francisco, CA 94117. Has aromatherapy kits and quality Aromatherapy education in the form of the Aromatherapy Studies Course. The home-study course is composed of 15 chapters with a study guide after each and sensory and essential oil experiments throughout.

Lebermuth. P.O. Box 4103. South Bend, IN 46634. Always a continuing source of quality essential oils, but remember to ask for their aromatherapy line as they also carry fragrance oils. Has a wonderful domestic Roman Chamomile oil.

Prima Fleur. 1525 East San Francisco Blvd. #16. San Rafael, CA 94901. Quality true aromatherapy products, custom product developers, lovely essential oils and true hydrosols. They support The Aromatic Plant Project©.

## Glossary

Axillary—organs such as flowers and buds, when they are found in the upper angle of the junction of a leaf with the stem.

Deciduous—describing woody perennial plants that shed their leaves before the winter or dry season. Various environmental factors influence the onset of leaf drop (day length, temperature, intensity of the light).

Ecology—the study of the relationship between living organisms and the living (biotic) and non-living (abiotic) factors in the environment.

Empyreumatic—having an odor of burnt organic matter as a result of decomposition at the high temperature of distillation.

Eponymous—bearing the name of the name or name giver. An eponymous scent is one where to describe the scent you use the name of the plant. For example: Peppermint EO smells like peppermint.

Facies—The general appearance or makeup of a natural group.

Glabrous—describing a surface that is devoid of hairs or other projections. Smooth.

Gum—any substance (natural or synthetic) that swells in water to form gels. Strictly speaking, gums are always water soluble. For example: Gum acacia, Gum tragacanth.

Gum Acacia (*Acacia senegal*) also called gum arabic. Water soluble and when dissolved in boiling water, clarifies and makes a very good adhesive that is used, among other things, to make scented beads and pomanders. The gum is edible, nutritive, and acts as a demulcent to sooth irritated mucous membranes. It is also an ingredient in medicinal compounds for diarrhea, dysentery, coughs and catarrh. The bark of the acacia plant is very rich in tannin. (Herbs & Things)

Resins are sometimes called gums. However, gums form solutions or "sols" with water, resins do not. Resins are insoluble in water.

The word "gum" is truly an herbal term, as gums are used in herbalism to make sticky solutions in cosmetics or to adhere dry ingredients together.

Gum resin—exude naturally from plants or trees. Consist of both a gum and a resin, sometimes with a small amount of EO. For example: Benzoin.

Indigenous—describing an organism that is native to an area, i.e. that has not been introduced from elsewhere.

Lysigenous—inter-cellular spaces, formed by the breaking down of adjoining cells.

Morphology—the study of form, particularly external structure.

Niche—the place and role occupied by an organism in a community, determined by its nutritional requirements, habitat, etc. Different species may occupy a similar niche in different areas.

Oleo-gum-resin—is a term to describe certain gums that are oily and resinous. Oleo (oily or fatty in nature or look) gum (partly soluble in water) resin (partly or wholly soluble in alcohol). Therefore, an oleo-gum-resin has a nature that is partially soluble in water and alcohol and looks oily. Consists mainly of oil, gum, and resin. For example: Myrrh, Frankincense, and Opopanax.

Oleo-resin—prepared or natural material. Exude from trees—trunks or barks. Sometimes they are prepared in the laboratory and form as an evaporation residue. Oleo-resin often contain "fixed" oils. Can be described with color, "clear, viscous, light-colored." For example: Copaiba balsam.

Ovule—the female gamete and its protective and nutritive tissue, which develops into the dispersal unit or seed after fertilization in seed plants (a structure that develops into a seed). Also occasionally used for vaginal suppositries or boluses.

Persistent—leaves that cling all winter, even though withered.

Resin—natural or prepared. Exude from trees or plants. Formed by nature. Some resins are prepared in the laboratory as oleo-resins. Resins are solid to semi-solid, amorphous. If they contain no water they are translucent. Odorless, not soluble in water. Can be described generally as products that are used as incense, such as Copal from Mexico and Amber. These only yield fragrance upon burning.

Resinoid—obtained from resins. Resins are solvent extracted, yielding an alcohol-soluble substance that is less dense, more sticky and liquid-like, called a Resinoid. Viscous liquids, semi-solid. In a perfectly prepared resinoid, the odiferous material or EO is left intact. Olibanum resinoid is typical. The Olibanum, or natural oleo-gum-resin has been made soluble for perfume use by the removal of the water-soluble gum. For example: Resinoid of Frankincense.

Rosin—prepared from resins. It is a translucent, friable resin that is obtained from the oleo-resin or the dead wood of Pine trees by the removal of the turpentine. For lacquers, paint, to rosin violin bows.

Schizocarp—a dry fruit that is derived from two or more one-seeded carpels that divide into one-seeded units at maturity.

Sessile—unstalked, as a leaf with no petiole or a stigma with no style.

Stomatiferous—leaves that are marked by minute, intercellular fissures in the epidermis that are flanked by guard cells (marked by small openings on the surface of a leaf, through which gaseous exchange takes place).

Topology—the history of a region as indicated by its topography, which is the description of a particular place by its physical features.

# References

## Chapter One

Allen, J. Coombes. *Dictionary of Plant Names*. Portland, OR: Timber Press, 1995.

Britton, Lord & Hon. Addison Brown. *An Illustrated Flora of the Northern United States and Canada,* Vol. II, New York: Dover Publications, 1970.

FLORA MANUALS, REGIONAL FLORAS OF WHOLE AREAS.

Fuller, H.J. & Tippo, O. *College Botany*, New York: Henry Holt & Co., 1948.

Harrington, H.D. & Durrell, L.W. *How to Identify Plants* (Plant taxonomy). Chicago: The Swallow Press, 1957.

Hichman, C. ed. *The Jepson Manual of Higher Plants of California*, San Francisco: Univ. of California Press, 1993.

Keator, Glenn. Leaflet. Summer 1998.

Kindschey, Ketly. *Medicinal Wild Plants of the Prairie*. Kansas City, Kansas: University Press of Kansas, 1982.

Mabberly, D.J. *The Plant Book*. Cambridge, England: Cambridge University Press, 1989.

Peterson, Roger Tory. *Peterson's Guide to the East Coast Wildflowers*. New York: Houghton Mifflin, 1992.

_____ *Jeanne Rose's Modern Herbal*. New York: Putnam Publishing Group, 1987.

_____ ed. Rose, Jeanne & Earle, Susan. *The World of Aromatherapy*. Berkeley,CA: Frog, Ltd., 1996

Schnaubelt, Kurt. *Medical Aromatherapy*. Berkeley, North Atlantic Books, 1998.

Smith, James Payne, Jr. *Vascular Plant Families.* Mad River Press, Inc., 1977.

Tutin, T.G., Haywood, V.H., Burges, N.A., Moore, M.S., Valentine, D.H., Walters, S.M., and Webb, D.A. Editors, *Flora Europaea* Vol. 4, Cambridge: Cambridge University Press, 1976.

## Chapter Two

Brown, Wilber Roland. *Composition of Scientific Words.* Washington D.C.: Smithsonian Constitution Press. 1978.

Coombes, Allen, J. Dictionary of Plant Names. Portland, OR: Timber Press, 1995.

Flannery, Michael J. Personal letter, 1998.

*Flora Indica,* current edition.

Giuliani, Charmain. *Taxonomy for Gardeners.* A class at Strybing Arboretum. February 1999. She helped me with many of the backgrounds of these names.

Gledhill D. *The Names of Plants.* Cambridge, England: Cambridge University Press. 1985.

Jaeger, Edmund C. *A Source-Book of Biological Names and Terms.* Springfield, IL: Charles C. Thomas, 1955.

Lewis, C.T. *Elementary Latin Dictionary.* Oxford, Great Britain: Clarendon Press. 1979.

Lewis, C.T. & Short, Charles. *A Latin Dictionary.* Oxford, England Clarendon Press. 1980.

Lloyd, John. *Origin and History of all the Pharmacopeial Vegetable Drugs.* Cincinnati: Caxton Press, 1921.

Mabberly, D.J. *The Plant Book.* Cambridge, England: Cambridge University Press, 1989.

## Chapter Five

Arctander, Steffen. *Perfume and Flavor Materials of Natural Origin.* Elizabeth, NJ: Steffen Arctander, 1960.

Bailey, Liberty Hyde & Ethel, Zoe. *Hortus Third.* New York: MacMillan Publishing Co., 1976.

Franchomme, P. & Penoel, Docteur D. *L'Aromatherapie Exactement.* Limoges, France: Roger Jollois Editeur, 1990.

Guenther, Ernest, Ph.D. *The Essential Oils*. Malabar, FL: Krieger Publishing Company 1976, original edition 1952. in VI volumes.

Rose, Jeanne. *The Aromatherapy Book: Applications & Inhalations*. Berkeley, CA: North Atlantic Books, 3rd. ed., 1994.

Suskind, Patrick. Perfume. New York, NY: Pocket Book, 1985.

Tutin, Haywood, Burges, Moore, Valentine, Walters and Webb, Editors, *Flora Europaea* Vol. 4, Cambridge: Cambridge University Press, 1976.

## Chapter Seven

Bailey, Liberty Hyde & Ethel, Zoe. *Hortus Third*. New York: MacMillan Publishing Co., 1976.

Balacs, Tony & Tisserand, Robert. *Essential Oil Safety: A Guide for Health Care Professionals.* New York: Churchill Livingstone, 1995.

Boulos, Loutfy. *Medicinal Plants of North Africa*. Algonac, MI: Reference Publishers, 1983.

Britton, Lord & Hon. Addison Brown. *An Illustrated Flora of the Northern United States and Canada,* Vol. II, New York: Dover Publications, 1970.

Clifford, Derek. *Pelargoniums*. Great Britain: Blandford Press, 1958.

Franchomme, P. & Penoel, Docteur D. *L'Aromatherapie Exactement*. Limoges, France: Roger Jollois Editeur, 1990.

Gerth, Van Wijk. *A Dictionary of Plant Names* Vol. 1. Amsterdam: A. Asher & Co., 1971.

Guenther, Ernest, Ph.D. *The Essential Oils*. Malabar, FL: Krieger Publishing Company 1976, original edition 1952. in VI volumes.

Khamis, Al-Said, Islam, Tariq, Parmar and Ageel, *Antifertility... extract of Cuminum cyminum.* Fitoterapia, 59, 5-9, 1988.

Harris, Thaddeus. *The Natural History of the Bible*. Ontario, Canada: Provoker Press, 1968.

Hornok, L. *Cultivation and Processing of Medicinal Plants*. Chichester, England: John Wiley & Sons, 1992.

Lawless, Julia. *The Encyclopedia of Essential Oils*. Massachusetts: Element, 1992.

Lawrence, Brian M. Monographs on Essential Oils. *Perfumer and Flavourist*. Carol Stream: Allured Publishing, 1975-94.

Lewis, Walter. & Memory, P.F. Elvin-Lewis. *Medical Botany: Plants Affecting Man's Health.* New York: John Wiley & Sons, 1977.

Mabberly, D.J. *The Plant Book.* Cambridge, England: Cambridge University Press, 1989.

Mann, John. *Murder, Magic, and Medicine.* New York: Oxford University Press, 1993.

Redell, Rayford. adapted from *The San Francisco Chronicle.* 1998.

Rimmel, Eugene. *The Book of Perfumes.* London: Chapman and Hall, 1865.

Rose, Jeanne. *The Aromatherapy Book: Applications & Inhalations.* Berkeley, CA: North Atlantic Books, 3rd. ed., 1994.

_____*Guide to [375] Essential Oils.* San Francisco, CA: Jeanne Rose Aromatherapy, 3rd ed., 1998.

_____*The Herbal Body Book.* New York: Grosset & Dunlap, 1976.

_____*The Aromatic Plant Project.* California: World of Aromatherapy Conference Proceedings, 1996.

Schultes, Richard Evans, Ed. *Medicines from the Earth: A Guide to Healing Plants.* Alfred Van Der Marck Editors, 1983.

Sudworth, George B. *Forest Trees of the Pacific Slope.* New York, NY: Dover Publications, 1967.

Tutin, Haywood, Burges, Moore, Valentine, Walters and Webb, Editors, *Flora Europaea* Vol. 4, Cambridge: Cambridge University Press, 1976.

Vincent, G. [Effect of limiting overall growth potential on the architectrue of rose geranium *(Pelargonium* sp.*)*.] Effet de la limitation du potentiel de croissance global sur l'architecture de Géranium Rosat *(Pelargonium* sp.*). Acta Botanica Gallica* (1995) 142 (5) 451-461 [Fr, en, 10 ref.] CIRAD-Réunion, Station de la Bretagne, 97487 Saint-Denis Cedex, Réunion.

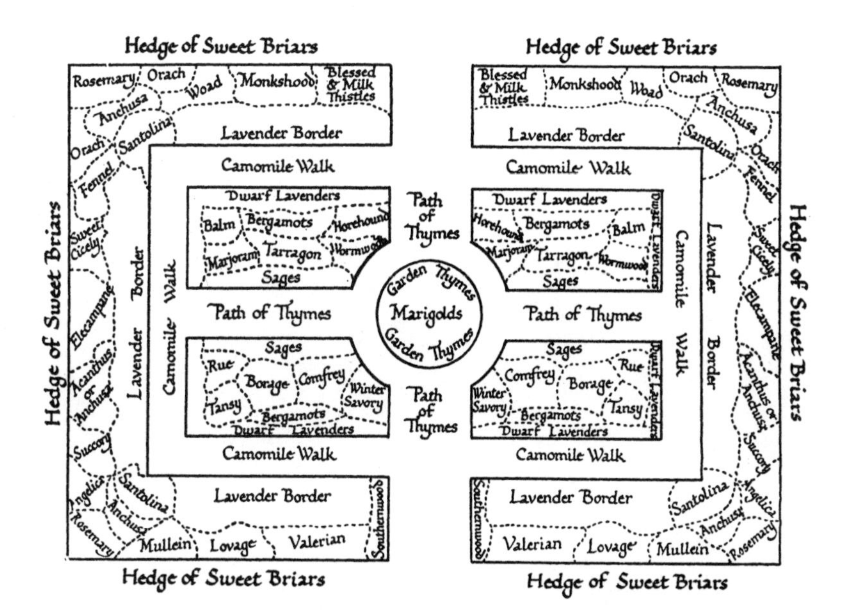
Hedge of Sweet Briars
Hedge of Sweet Briars
Rosemary
Orach
Woad
Monkshood
Blessed & Milk Thistles
Anchusa
Santolina
Lavender Border
Orach
Fennel
Sweet Cicely
Elecampane
Acanthus or Anchusa
Succory
Angelica
Santolina
Anchusa
Rosemary
Mullein
Lovage
Valerian
Southernwood
Lavender Border
Camomile Walk
Dwarf Lavenders
Balm
Bergamots
Horehound
Marjoram
Tarragon
Wormwood
Sages
Path of Thymes
Path of Thymes
Garden Thymes
Marigolds
Garden Thymes
Sages
Rue
Borage
Comfrey
Winter Savory
Tansy
Bergamots
Dwarf Lavenders
Path of Thymes
Camomile Walk
Lavender Border
Camomile Walk
Hedge of Sweet Briars
Blessed & Milk Thistles
Monkshood
Woad
Orach
Rosemary
Anchusa
Santolina
Orach
Fennel
Lavender Border
Camomile Walk
Dwarf Lavenders
Horehound
Bergamots
Balm
Marjoram
Tarragon
Wormwood
Sages
Path of Thymes
Sages
Rue
Comfrey
Borage
Winter Savory
Tansy
Bergamots
Dwarf Lavenders
Dwarf Lavenders
Dwarf Lavenders
Camomile Walk
Lavender Border
Sweet Cicely
Elecampane
Acanthus or Anchusa
Succory
Camomile Walk
Lavender Border
Santolina
Angelica
Anchusa
Rosemary
Southernwood
Valerian
Lovage
Mullein
Hedge of Sweet Briars
Hedge of Sweet Briars
Hedge of Sweet Briars

# Bibliography

Allen, J. Coombes. *Dictionary of Plant Names*. Portland, OR: Timber Press, 1995.

Arctander, Steffen. *Perfume and Flavor Materials of Natural Origin.* Elizabeth, NJ: Steffen Arctander, 1960.

Bailey, Liberty Hyde & Ethel, Zoe. *Hortus Third.* New York: MacMillan Publishing Co., 1976.

Balacs, Tony & Tisserand, Robert. *Essential Oil Safety: A Guide for Health Care Professionals.* New York: Churchill Livingstone, 1995.

Boulos, Loutfy. *Medicinal Plants of North Africa.* Algonac, MI: Reference Publishers, 1983.

Britton, Lord & Hon. Addison Brown. *An Illustrated Flora of the Northern United States and Canada,* Vol. II, New York: Dover Publications, 1970.

Clifford, Derek. *Pelargoniums.* Great Britain: Blandford Press, 1958.

FLORA MANUALS, REGIONAL FLORAS OF WHOLE AREAS.

Franchomme, P. & Penoel, Docteur D. *L'Aromatherapie Exactement.* Limoges, France: Roger Jollois Editeur, 1990.

Fuller, H.J. & Tippo, O. *College Botany*, New York: Henry Holt & Co., 1948.

Gerth, Van Wijk. *A Dictionary of Plant Names* Vol. 1. Amsterdam: A. Asher & Co., 1971.

*Gray's* Manual of Flowering Plants of the Northeastern United States.

Guenther, Ernest, Ph.D. *The Essential Oils.* Malabar, FL: Krieger Publishing Company 1976, original edition 1952. in VI volumes.

Harrington, H.D. & Durrell, L.W. *How to Identify Plants* (Plant taxonomy). Chicago: The Swallow Press, 1957.

Harris, Thaddeus. *The Natural History of the Bible.* Ontario, Canada: Provoker Press, 1968.

Hichman, C. ed. *The Jepson Manual of Higher Plants of California*, San Francisco: Univ. of California Press, 1993.

Hornok, L. *Cultivation and Processing of Medicinal Plants*. Chichester, England: John Wiley & Sons, 1992.

Jaeger, Edmund C. *A Source-Book of Biological Names and Terms*. Springfield, IL: Charles C. Thomas, 1955.

Keator, Glenn. Leaflet. Summer 1998.

Kindschey, Ketly. *Medicinal Wild Plants of the Prairie*. Kansas City, Kansas: University Press of Kansas, 1982.

Lawless, Julia. *The Encyclopedia of Essential Oils*. Massachusetts: Element, 1992.

Lawrence, Brian M. Monographs on Essential Oils. *Perfumer and Flavourist*. Carol Stream: Allured Publishing, 1975-94.

Lewis, Walter. & Memory, P.F. Elvin-Lewis. *Medical Botany: Plants Affecting Man's Health*. New York: John Wiley & Sons, 1977.

Lloyd, John. *Origin and History of all the Pharmacopeial Vegetable Drugs*. Cincinnati: Caxton Press, 1921.

Mabberly, D.J. *The Plant Book*. Cambridge, England: Cambridge University Press, 1989.

Mann, John. *Murder, Magic, and Medicine*. New York: Oxford University Press, 1993.

Peterson, Roger Tory. *Peterson's Guide to the East Coast Wildflowers*. New York: Houghton Mifflin, 1992.

Redell, Rayford. adapted from *The San Francisco Chronicle*. 1998.

Rimmel, Eugene. *The Book of Perfumes*. London: Chapman and Hall, 1865.

Rose, Jeanne. *The Aromatherapy Book: Applications & Inhalations*. Berkeley, CA: North Atlantic Books, 3rd. ed., 1994.

_____*The Aromatic Plant Project*. California: World of Aromatherapy Conference Proceedings, 1996.

_____*Guide to [225] Essential Oils*. San Francisco, CA: Jeanne Rose Aromatherapy, 3rd edition, 1994.

_____*Guide to [375] Essential Oils*. San Francisco, CA: Jeanne Rose Aromatherapy, 3rd ed., 1998.

_____*The Herbal Body Book*. New York: Grosset & Dunlap, 1976.

_____*Jeanne Rose's Modern Herbal*. New York: Putnam Publishing Group, 1987.

_____ed. Rose, Jeanne & Earle, Susan. *The World of Aromatherapy.* Berkeley, CA: Frog, Ltd., 1996.

Schnaubelt, Kurt. *Medical Aromatherapy.* Berkeley, North Atlantic Books, 1998.

Schultes, Richard Evans, Ed. *Medicines from the Earth: A Guide to Healing Plants.* Alfred Van Der Marck Editors, 1983.

Smith, James Payne, Jr. *Vascular Plant Families.* Mad River Press, Inc., 1977.

Sudworth, George B. *Forest Trees of the Pacific Slope.* New York, NY: Dover Publications, 1967.

Suskind, Patrick. Perfume. New York, NY: Pocket Book, 1985.

Tutin, Haywood, Burges, Moore, Valentine, Walters and Webb, Editors, *Flora Europaea* Vol. 4, Cambridge: Cambridge University Press, 1976.

Vincent, G. [Effect of limiting overall growth potential on the architectrue of rose geranium *(Pelargonium* sp.*)*.] Effet de la limitation du potentiel de croissance global sur l'architecture de Géranium Rosat *(Pelargonium* sp.*)*. *Acta Botanica Gallica* (1995) 142 (5) 451-461 [Fr, en, 10 ref.] CIRAD-Réunion, Station de la Bretagne, 97487 Saint-Denis Cedex, Réunion.

# Index